Diabetes
FOR
DUMMIES
POCKET EDITION

by Alan L. Rubin, MD

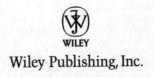

WILEY

Wiley Publishing, Inc.

Diabetes For Dummies,® Pocket Edition

Published by
Wiley Publishing, Inc.
111 River St.
Hoboken, NJ 07030-5774
www.wiley.com

For general information on our other products and services, please contact our Customer Care Department within the U.S. at 877-762-2974, outside the U.S. at 317-572-3993, or fax 317-572-4002.

For technical support, please visit www.wiley.com/techsupport.

Wiley also publishes its books in a variety of electronic formats. Some content that appears in print may not be available in electronic books.

ISBN: 978-0-470-91590-5

Manufactured in the United States of America

10 9 8 7 6 5 4 3 2 1

Publisher's Acknowledgments

Project Editor: Traci Cumbay
Composition Services: Indianapolis Composition Services Department
Cover Photo: © Purestock

WILEY

Table of Contents

Introduction

What's funny about diabetes? It's a disease, isn't it? Sure, it's a disease, but the people who have it at the beginning of the 21st century are the most fortunate group in history.

It reminds me of the story of the doctor who called his patient to give him the results of his blood tests. "I have bad news and worse news," said the doctor.

"My gosh," said the patient, "What's the bad news?"

"Your lab tests indicate that you have only 24 hours to live," said the doctor.

"What could be worse than that?" said the patient.

"I've been trying to reach you since yesterday," said the doctor.

Those of you with diabetes have a decade or more in which to avoid the long-term complications of this disease. In a sense, a diagnosis of diabetes is both good news and bad news. It is bad news because you have a disease you would happily do without. It is good news if you use it to make some changes in your lifestyle that can not only prevent complications but help you to live a longer and higher-quality life.

As for laughing about it, at times you will feel like doing anything but laughing. But scientific studies are clear about the benefits of a positive attitude. In a very few words: He who laughs, lasts. Another point is that people learn more and retain more when humor is part of the process.

If you have experienced something funny during the course of your diabetes care, I hope you share it with me. My goal is not to trivialize human suffering by being comic about it, but to lighten the burden of a chronic disease by showing that it is not all gloom and doom.

Many of you have shared your stories with me, permitting me to laugh and cry with you. One of the best is the following from Andrea in Canada:

> *My 3-year-old daughter was recently diagnosed with diabetes type one. It has been a rough time. To help us out my brother and his wife bought us your book, Diabetes For Dummies. One day my daughter saw this bright yellow book and asked what I was reading. I told her Diabetes For Dummies. As soon as the words came out of my mouth, I regretted it. I didn't want her to think that dummies got diabetes so I quickly added, "I am the dummy." Without missing a beat, she then asked, "Am I the diabetes?"*

> *The story doesn't just end there. The other day she was relaxing on the couch. She looked at me and said, "I don't want to have diabetes anymore." Feeling terrible I responded, "I know sweetie; I don't want you to have it anymore either." I then explained that she would have diabetes for the rest of her life. With a very concerned look she then asked, "Will you be the dummy for the rest of your life?"*

*As sad as it is, I guess you're right, **one must look for humor in everything**, otherwise we would have broken down by now.*

About This Book

You're not required to read this book from cover to cover, although if you know nothing about diabetes, that may be a good approach. This book is designed to serve as a source for information about the problems that arise over the years. You can find the latest facts about diabetes and the best sources to discover any information that comes out after the publication of this edition.

Conventions Used in This Book

Diabetes is all about sugar. But sugars come in many types. So doctors avoid using the words *sugar* and *glucose* interchangeably. In this book (unless I slip up), I use the word *glucose* rather than *sugar*.

Foolish Assumptions

The book assumes that you know nothing about diabetes. You will not suddenly have to face a term that is not explained and that you never heard of before. For those who already know a lot about diabetes, you can find more in-depth explanations. You can pick and choose how much you want to know about a subject, but the key points are clearly marked.

Icons Used in This Book

The icons alert you to information you must know, information you should know, and information you may find interesting but can live without.

 When you see this icon, it means the information is essential and you should be aware of it.

 This icon points out when you should see your doctor (for example, if your blood glucose level is too high or you need a particular test done).

 This icon marks important information that can save you time and energy.

 This icon warns against potential problems (for example, if you don't treat a complication of diabetes properly).

Where to Go from Here

Where you go from here depends on your needs. You're welcome to read straight through or to skip around the book, reading whatever interests you or addresses your questions.

If you want even more information on diabetes, from the complications of the disease to picking out the right doctor for you to managing diabetes through lifestyle changes, check out the full-size version of *Diabetes For Dummies,* 3rd Edition (Wiley). Simply head to your local bookseller or go to www. dummies.com.

As my mother used to say when she gave me a present, use this book in good health.

Chapter 1

Getting the Lowdown on Diabetes

- -

In This Chapter

▶ Meeting others with diabetes

▶ Understanding prediabetes

▶ Finding out what diabetes does

▶ Coping with the initial diagnosis

▶ Upholding your quality of life

▶ Finding help when coping is tough

- -

As a person with diabetes, you are more than the sum of your blood glucose levels. You have feelings, and you have a history. The way that you respond to the challenges of diabetes determines whether the disease will be a moderate annoyance or the source of major sickness. In this chapter, I show you how diabetes affects not just your body but your heart and mind.

You Are Not Alone

Are you as pretty as Nicole Johnson, the 1999 Miss America? Are you as funny as Jackie Gleason or Jack Benny? Are you an actor with the talent of James Cagney, Spencer Tracy, or Elizabeth Taylor? Can you hit a tennis ball like Arthur Ashe? Can you paint like Paul Cézanne? Do you have the charisma of Gamel Abdel-Nasser? Can you write like Ernest Hemingway or H. G. Wells? Can you sing like Ella Fitzgerald or Elvis Presley? Do you have the inventive powers of Thomas Alva Edison? You have at least one thing in common with all of these famous people. That's right — diabetes.

The list of people with diabetes who have achieved greatness is long. I emphasize this point because I want to drive home another: *Diabetes shouldn't stop you from doing what you want to do with your life.* You must follow the rules of good diabetic care, but if you follow these rules, you will actually be healthier than people without diabetes who smoke, overeat, and/or don't exercise enough.

 If you follow the rules of good diabetes care, you will be just as healthy as a person without diabetes.

Perhaps the many people with diabetes who have achieved greatness used the same personal strengths to overcome the difficulties associated with diabetes and to excel at their particular callings. Or maybe their diabetes forced them to be stronger and to persevere more, which contributed to their success.

You find few areas (such as piloting a commercial flight) in which certain people with diabetes can't participate — due to the ignorance of some legislators. These last few blocks to complete freedom of choice for those with diabetes will come down as you show that you can safely and competently do anything that a person without diabetes can do.

Detecting Prediabetes

Diabetes doesn't suddenly appear one day with no previous notification by your body. For a period of time, which may last up to ten years, you don't quite achieve the criteria for a diagnosis of diabetes, but you aren't quite normal either. During this time, you have what's called *prediabetes.*

A person with prediabetes doesn't usually develop eye disease, kidney disease, or nerve damage (all potential complications of diabetes). However, this person's risk of developing heart disease and brain attacks is much greater than the risk for someone with entirely normal blood glucose levels. Prediabetes has a lot in common with insulin resistance syndrome, also known as the *metabolic syndrome.*

 Between 20 and 30 million people in the United States have prediabetes, although most don't know it. Testing for prediabetes is a good idea for everyone over the age of 45. I also recommend testing for people who are under 45 if they're overweight and have one or more of the following risk factors:

✔ Being part of a high-risk ethnic group: African American, Hispanic, Asian, or Native American

✔ High blood pressure

✔ Low HDL or "good" cholesterol

✔ High triglycerides

✔ A family history of diabetes

✔ Diabetes during a pregnancy or a newborn who weighed more than nine pounds

Testing for prediabetes involves finding out your
blood glucose level — the level of sugar in your blood.
Prediabetes exists when the body's blood glucose
level is higher than normal but not high enough to
meet the standard definition of diabetes mellitus
(which I discuss in the section "Testing for diabetes,"
later in this chapter). Table 1-1 shows the glucose
levels that indicate prediabetes.

Table 1-1	Diagnosing Prediabetes	
Condition	*Glucose Before Eating*	*Glucose One Hour After Eating*
Normal	Less than 100 mg/dl (5.5 mmol/L)	Less than 140 mg/dl (7.8 mmol/L)
Prediabetes	100–126 mg/dl (5.5–7 mmol/L)	140–199 mg/dl 7.8–11.1 mmol/L

Diagnosing prediabetes is crucial because lifestyle changes, especially diet and exercise, have
been shown to prevent the onset of diabetes in
people with prediabetes. For those who don't
respond to lifestyle changes, medication may
accomplish the same thing.

Understanding What Diabetes Does

When prediabetes becomes diabetes, the body's
blood glucose level is even higher. In this section,
I discuss the role of glucose in your body, how to test
for diabetes, and the symptoms you may experience
associated with diabetes.

Recognizing the role of glucose

Many different sugars exist in nature, but glucose is the sugar that has the starring role in the body, providing a source of instant energy so that muscles can move and important chemical reactions can take place. Sugar is a carbohydrate, one of three sources of energy in the body. The other sources are protein and fat.

Table sugar, or *sucrose*, is actually two different kinds of sugar — glucose and fructose — linked together. Fructose is the type of sugar found in fruits and vegetables. It is sweeter than glucose, which means that sucrose is sweeter than glucose as well. Your taste buds require less sucrose or fructose to get the same sweetening power of glucose.

Testing for diabetes

The standard definition of diabetes mellitus is excessive glucose in a blood sample. For years, doctors set this level fairly high. The standard level for a normal glucose was lowered in 1997 because too many people were experiencing complications of diabetes even though they didn't have the disease by the then-current standard. In November 2003, the standard level was modified again.

After much discussion, many meetings, and the usual deliberations that surround a momentous decision, the American Diabetes Association published the new standard for diagnosis, which includes any one of the following three criteria:

  ✔ **Casual plasma glucose** concentration greater than or equal to 200 mg/dl, along with symptoms of diabetes (which I discuss in the section "Losing control of glucose" later in this chapter). Casual plasma glucose refers to your glucose level when you eat normally prior to the test.

Mg/dl stands for *milligrams per deciliter*. The rest of the world uses the International System (SI), where the units are mmol/L, which means *millimoles per liter*. To get mmol/L, you divide mg/dl by 18. Therefore, 200 mg/dl equals 11.1 mmol/L.

✔ **Fasting plasma glucose (FPG)** of greater than or equal to 126 mg/dl or 7 mmol/L. *Fasting* means that you have consumed no food for eight hours prior to the test.

✔ **Blood glucose** of greater than or equal to 200 mg/dl (11.1 mmol/L) when tested two hours (2-h PG) after ingesting 75 grams of glucose by mouth. This test has long been known as the *Oral Glucose Tolerance Test*. Although this test is rarely done because it takes time and is cumbersome, it remains the gold standard for the diagnosis of diabetes.

Putting it another way:

✔ FPG less than 100 mg/dl (5.5 mmol/L) is a normal fasting glucose.

✔ FPG greater than or equal to 100 mg/dl but less than 126 mg/dl (7.0 mmol/L) is impaired fasting glucose (indicating prediabetes).

✔ FPG equal to or greater than 126 mg/dl (7.0 mmol/L) gives a provisional diagnosis of diabetes.

✔ 2-h PG less than 140 mg/dl (7.8 mmol/L) is normal glucose tolerance.

✔ 2-h PG greater than or equal to 140 mg/dl but less than 200 mg/dl (11.1 mmol/L) is impaired glucose tolerance.

✔ 2-h PG equal to or greater than 200 mg/dl gives a provisional diagnosis of diabetes.

Testing positive for diabetes one time is not enough to confirm a diagnosis. Any one of the tests must be positive on another occasion to make a diagnosis of diabetes. I've had patients come to me with a diagnosis of diabetes after being tested only once, and a second test has shown the initial diagnosis to be incorrect.

Controlling glucose

In order to understand the symptoms of diabetes, you need to know a little about the way the body normally handles glucose and what happens when things go wrong.

A hormone called *insulin* (see Chapter 2) finely controls the level of glucose in your blood. A *hormone* is a chemical substance made in one part of the body that travels (usually through the bloodstream) to a distant part of the body where it performs its work. In the case of insulin, that work is to act like a key to open the inside of a cell (such as a muscle, a fat, or other cell) so that glucose can enter. If glucose can't enter the cell, it can provide no energy to the body.

Insulin is essential for growth. In addition to providing the key to entry of glucose into the cell, insulin is considered the *builder hormone* because it enables fat and muscle to form. It promotes the storage of glucose in a form called *glycogen* for use when fuel is not coming in. It also blocks the breakdown of protein. Without insulin, you do not survive for long.

With this fine-tuning, your body keeps the level of glucose pretty steady at about 60 to 100 mg/dl (3.3 to 5.5 mmol/L) all the time.

Losing control of glucose

Your glucose starts to rise in your blood when you don't have a sufficient amount of insulin or when your insulin is not working effectively. When your glucose rises above 180 mg/dl (10.0 mmol/L), glucose begins to spill into the urine and make it sweet. Up to that point, the kidney, the filter for the blood, is able to extract the glucose before it enters your urine. The loss of glucose into the urine leads to many of the short-term complications of diabetes.

The following list contains the most common early symptoms of diabetes and how they occur. One or more of the following symptoms may be present when diabetes is diagnosed:

- ✔ **Frequent urination and thirst:** The glucose in the urine draws more water out of your blood, so more urine forms. More urine in your bladder makes you feel the need to urinate more frequently, day and night. As the amount of water in your blood declines, you feel thirsty and drink much more frequently.

- ✔ **Fatigue:** Without sufficient insulin, or if the insulin is not effective, glucose can't be used as a fuel to move muscles or to facilitate the many other chemical reactions that have to take place to produce energy. A person with diabetes often complains of fatigue and feels much stronger after treatment allows glucose to enter her cells again.

- ✔ **Weight loss:** Weight loss occurs among some people with diabetes because they lack insulin. When insulin is lacking for any reason, the body begins to break down. You lose muscle tissue. Some of the muscle converts into glucose even though it cannot get into cells. It passes out of your body in the urine. Fat tissue breaks down into small fat particles that can provide an alternate source of energy. As your body breaks down and you lose glucose in the urine, you often experience weight loss. However, most people with diabetes are heavy rather than skinny.

✔ **Persistent vaginal infection among women:** As blood glucose rises, all the fluids in your body contain higher levels of glucose, including the sweat and body secretions such as semen in men and vaginal secretions in women. Many bugs, such as bacteria and fungi, thrive in the high-glucose environment. Women begin to complain of itching or burning, an abnormal discharge from the vagina, and sometimes an odor.

Reacting to Your Diagnosis

Do you remember what you were doing when you found out that you had diabetes? Unless you were too young to understand, the news was quite a shock. Suddenly you had a condition from which people die. Many of the feelings that you went through were exactly those of a person learning that he or she is dying. The following sections describe the normal stages of reacting to a diagnosis of a major medical condition such as diabetes.

Experiencing denial

Your first response was probably to deny that you had diabetes, despite all the evidence. Your doctor may have helped you to deny by saying that you had just "a touch of diabetes," which is an impossibility equivalent to "a touch of pregnancy." You probably looked for any evidence that the whole thing was a mistake.

Ultimately, you had to accept the diagnosis and begin to gather the information you needed to help yourself. When you accepted the diabetes diagnosis, I hope you also shared the news with your family, friends, and people close to you. Having diabetes isn't something to be ashamed of, and you shouldn't hide it from anyone. When you're accepting and open about having diabetes, you'll find that you're far from alone in your situation.

You need the help of everyone in your environment, from your co-workers who need to know not to tempt you with treats that you can't eat, to your friends who need to know how to give you *glucagon,* a treatment for low blood glucose, if you become unconscious from a severe insulin reaction.

Your diabetes isn't your fault — nor is it a form of leprosy or some other disease that carries a social stigma. Diabetes also isn't contagious; no one can catch it from you.

One of my patients told me about experiences she had that helped her feel part of a community. She arrived at work one morning and was very worried when she realized that she'd forgotten her insulin. But she quickly found a source of comfort when she remembered that she could go to a diabetic co-worker and ask to borrow some insulin. Another time, she was at a party and stepped into a friend's bedroom to take a shot of insulin, and she found a man there doing the same thing.

Feeling anger

When you've passed the stage of denying that you have diabetes, you may become angry that you're saddled with this "terrible" diagnosis. But you'll quickly find that diabetes isn't so terrible and that

you can't do anything to rid yourself of the disease.
Anger only worsens your situation.

 As long as you're angry, you are not in a prob-
lem-solving mode. Diabetes requires your focus
and attention. Use your energy positively — to
find creative ways to manage your diabetes.

Bargaining for more time

The stage of anger often transitions into a stage when
you become increasingly aware of the loss of immor-
tality and begin to bargain for more time. Even though
you probably realize that you have plenty of life
ahead of you, you may feel overwhelmed by the talk
of complications, blood tests, and pills or insulin. You
may experience depression, which makes good diabetic care all the more difficult.

Studies have shown that people with diabetes suffer
from depression at a rate that is two to four times
higher than the rate for the general population. Those
with diabetes also experience anxiety at a rate three
to five times higher than people without diabetes.

If you suffer from depression, you may feel that your
diabetic situation creates problems for you that jus-
tify being depressed. You may rationalize your
depression in the following ways:

✔ Diabetes hinders you as you try to make friends.

✔ As a person with diabetes, you don't have the
freedom to choose your leisure activities.

✔ You may feel that you're too tired to overcome
difficulties.

✔ You may dread the future and possible diabetic
complications.

✔ You don't have the freedom to eat what you want.

✔ All the minor inconveniences of dealing with diabetes may produce a constant level of annoyance.

All the preceding concerns are legitimate, but they also are surmountable. How do you handle your many concerns and fend off depression? The following are a few important methods:

✔ Try to achieve excellent blood glucose control.

✔ Begin a regular exercise program.

✔ Tell a friend or relative how you're feeling; get it off your chest.

✔ Recognize that every abnormal blip in your blood glucose is not your fault.

Moving on

If you can't overcome the depression brought on by your diabetic concerns, you may need to consider therapy or antidepressant drugs. But you probably won't reach that point. You may experience the various stages of reacting to your diabetes in a different order than I describe in the previous sections. Some stages may be more prominent, and others may be hardly noticeable.

Don't feel that any anger, denial, or depression is wrong. These are natural coping mechanisms that serve a psychological purpose for a brief time. Allow yourself to have these feelings — and then drop them. Move on and learn to live normally with your diabetes.

Maintaining a High Quality of Life

You may assume that a chronic disease like diabetes leads to a diminished quality of life. But must this be the case? Several studies have been done to evaluate this question.

The importance of taking control

One study, which lasted only 12 weeks, was described in the *Journal of the American Medical Association* in November 1998; it looked at the difference in the perceived quality of life between a group that had good diabetic control and a group that had poor diabetic control.

The well-controlled group had lower distress from symptoms, a perception that they were in better health, and a feeling that they could think and learn more easily. This translated into greater productivity, less absenteeism, and fewer days of restricted activity.

Most of the other studies of quality of life for people with diabetes have been long-term studies. In one study of more than 2,000 people with diabetes who were receiving many different levels of intensity of treatment, the overall response was that quality of life was lower for the person with diabetes than for the general population. But several factors separated those with the lower quality of life from those who expressed more contentment with life.

One factor that contributed to a lower quality of life rating was a lack of physical activity. This is one negative factor that you can alter immediately.

The (minimal) impact of insulin treatments

Perhaps you're afraid that intensified insulin treatment, which involves three or four daily shots of insulin and frequent testing of blood glucose, will keep you from doing the things that you want to do and will diminish your daily quality of life.

A study discussed in *Diabetes Care* in November 1998 explored whether the extra effort and time consumed by such diabetes treatments had an adverse effect on people's quality of life. The study compared people with diabetes to people with other chronic diseases, such as gastrointestinal disease and hepatitis (liver infection), and then compared all of those groups to a group of people who had no disease.

The diabetic group reported a higher quality of life than the other chronic illness groups. The people in the diabetic group were not so much concerned with the physical problems of diabetes, such as intense and time-consuming tests and treatments, as they were concerned with the social and psychological difficulties.

Other key quality-of-life factors

Many other studies have examined the different aspects of diabetes that affect quality of life. The following studies had some useful findings:

- **Family support:** People with diabetes greatly benefit from their families' help in dealing with their disease. But do people with diabetes in a close family have better diabetic control? One study in *Diabetes Care* in February 1998 attempted to answer this question and found some unexpected results.

Having a supportive family didn't necessarily mean that the person with diabetes would maintain better glucose control. But a supportive family did make the person with diabetes feel more physically capable in general and much more comfortable with his or her place in society.

✔ **Insulin injections for adults:** Do adults with diabetes who require insulin shots experience a diminished quality of life? A report in *Diabetes Care* in June 1998 found that insulin injections don't reduce the quality of life; the person's sense of physical and emotional well-being remains the same after beginning insulin injections as it was before injections were necessary.

✔ **Insulin injections for teenagers:** Teenagers who require insulin injections don't always accept the treatment as well as adults do, so teenagers more often experience a diminished quality of life.

However, a study of more than 2,000 teenagers in *Diabetes Care* in November 2001 showed that as their diabetic control improved, they experienced greater satisfaction with their lives and felt in better health, while they believed themselves to be less of a burden to their families.

✔ **Stress management:** A study described in *Diabetes Care* in January 2002 showed that lowering stress lowers blood glucose. Patients were divided into two groups, one of which received diabetes education alone and the other diabetes education plus five sessions of stress management. The latter group showed significant improvement in diabetic control compared to those who received only diabetes education.

✔ **Quality of life over the long term:** How does a person's perception of quality of life change over time? As they age, do most people with diabetes feel that their quality of life increases, decreases, or persists at a steady level?

The consensus of studies is that most people with diabetes experience an increasing quality of life as they get older. People feel better about themselves and their diabetes after dealing with the disease for a decade or more. This is the healing property of time.

The bottom line

Putting all the information in the previous sections together, what can you do to maintain a high quality of life with diabetes?

Here are the steps that accomplish the most for you:

✔ Keep your blood glucose as normal as possible.

✔ Make exercise a regular part of your lifestyle.

✔ Get plenty of support from family, friends, and medical resources.

✔ Stay aware of the latest developments in diabetes care.

✔ Maintain a healthy attitude. Remember that someday you will laugh about things that bug you now, so why wait?

When You're Having Trouble Coping

You wouldn't hesitate to seek help for your physical ailments associated with diabetes, but you may be reluctant to seek help when you can't adjust psychologically to diabetes. The problem is that sooner or later, your psychological maladjustment will ruin any control that you have over your diabetes. And, of course, you won't lead a very pleasant life if you're in a depressed or anxious state all the time.

 You may be past the point of handling your diabetes on your own and may be suffering from depression if you:

✔ Can't sleep

✔ Have no energy when you're awake

✔ Can't think clearly

✔ Can't find activities that interest or amuse you

✔ Feel worthless

✔ Have frequent thoughts of suicide

✔ Have no appetite

✔ Find no humor in anything

If you recognize several of these symptoms as features of your daily life, you need to get some help. Your sense of hopelessness may include the feeling that no one else can help you — and that simply isn't true.

Your primary physician or endocrinologist is the first place to go for advice. He or she may help you to see the need for some short-term or long-term therapy. Well-trained therapists — especially therapists who are trained to take care of people with diabetes — can see solutions that you can't see in your current state. You need to find a therapist whom you can trust, so that when you're feeling low you can talk to this person and feel assured that he or she is very interested in your welfare.

Your therapist may decide that you would benefit from medication to treat the anxiety or depression. Currently, many drugs are available that are proven safe and free of side effects. Sometimes a brief period of medication is enough to help you adjust to your diabetes.

 You can also find help in a support group. The huge and continually growing number of support groups shows that positive things are happening in these groups. In most support groups, participants share their stories and problems, which helps everyone involved cope with their own feelings of isolation, futility, or depression.

Chapter 2

Understanding Types of Diabetes

- -

In This Chapter

▶ Paying attention to your pancreas

▶ Comparing type 1 and type 2 diabetes

▶ Investigating gestational diabetes

▶ Being aware of other types of diabetes

- -

*H*ere's the good news: You can prevent diabetes. Here's the bad news: You can't do so quite as easily as you may like. Your best method for preventing diabetes is to pick your parents carefully, but that method is slightly impractical, even with modern technology.

This chapter shows you how to identify whether you're at risk for type 1 or type 2 diabetes, and it covers definite actions that you can take to prevent both of these types of diabetes. This chapter also helps you get a clear understanding of your type of diabetes, how it relates to the other types of diabetes, and how the failure of your friendly pancreas to do its assigned job can lead to a host of unfortunate consequences.

Getting to Know Your Pancreas

Ladies and gentlemen, I'd like to introduce you to
your pancreas. This shy little organ — which you've
probably never given a moment's attention — hides
behind your stomach quietly doing its work, assisting
with digestion first and then helping to make use of
the digested food.

The pancreas has two major functions. One is to produce *digestive enzymes,* which are the chemicals in
your small intestine that help to break down food.
Your pancreas's other function is to produce and
secrete directly into the blood a hormone of major
importance, *insulin.*

If you understand only one hormone in your
body, insulin should be that hormone (especially if you want to understand diabetes). Over
the course of your life, the insulin that your
body produces or the insulin that you inject into
your body affects whether you control your diabetes and avoid the complications of the
disease.

Think of your insulin as an insurance agent, who lives
in San Francisco (which is your pancreas) but travels
from there to do business in Seattle (your muscles),
Denver (your fat tissue), Los Angeles (your liver), and
other places. This insulin insurance agent is insuring
your good health.

Wherever insulin travels in your body, it opens up the
cells so that glucose can enter them. After glucose
enters, the cells can immediately use it for energy,
store it in a storage form of glucose (called *glycogen*)
for rapid use later on, or convert it to fat for use even
later as energy.

After glucose leaves your blood and enters your cells, your blood glucose level falls. Your pancreas can tell when your glucose is falling, and it turns off the release of insulin to prevent unhealthy low levels of blood glucose called *hypoglycemia*. At the same time, your liver begins to release glucose from storage and makes new glucose from amino acids in your blood.

If your insurance agent (insulin, remember?) doesn't show up when you need him (meaning that you have an absence of insulin, as in type 1 diabetes) or he does a poor job when he shows up (such as when you have a resistance to insulin, as in type 2 diabetes), your blood glucose may start to climb. High blood glucose is the beginning of all your problems.

Doctors have proven that high blood glucose is bad for you and that keeping the blood glucose as normal as possible prevents the complications of diabetes. Most treatments for diabetes are directed at restoring the blood glucose to normal.

Considering Type 1 Diabetes

The following sections detail the symptoms and causes of *type 1 diabetes mellitus,* which used to be called *juvenile diabetes* or *insulin-dependent diabetes.*

Identifying symptoms of type 1 diabetes

Following are some of the major signs and symptoms of type 1 diabetes. If you experience the following symptoms, ask your doctor about the possibility that you have diabetes:

✔ **Frequent urination:** You experience frequent urination because your kidneys can't return all the glucose to your bloodstream when your blood glucose level is greater than 180 mg/dl (10 mmol/L). The large amount of glucose in your urine makes the urine very concentrated. As a result, your body draws water out of your blood and into the urine to reduce that high concentration of glucose. This water and glucose fill up the bladder repeatedly.

✔ **Increase in thirst:** Your thirst increases as you experience frequent urination because you lose so much water in the urine that your body begins to dehydrate.

✔ **Weight loss:** You lose weight as your body loses glucose in the urine and your body breaks down muscle and fat looking for energy.

✔ **Increase in hunger:** Your body has plenty of extra glucose in the blood, but your cells become malnourished because you lack insulin to allow the glucose to enter your cells. As a result, you become increasingly hungry. Your body goes through "hunger in the midst of plenty."

✔ **Weakness:** You feel weak because your muscle cells and other tissues do not get the energy that they require from glucose.

Type 1 diabetes used to be called *juvenile diabetes* because it occurs most frequently in children. However, so many cases are found in adults that doctors don't use the term *juvenile* any more. Some children are diagnosed early in life, and other children have a more severe onset of the disease as they get a little older.

With older children, the early signs and symptoms of diabetes may have been missed by parents, counselors, or teachers. These kids have a great deal of fat breakdown in their bodies to provide energy, and this fat breakdown creates other problems. *Ketone bodies,* products of the breakdown of fats, begin to accumulate in the blood and spill into the urine. Ketone bodies are acidic and lead to nausea, abdominal pain, and sometimes vomiting.

At the same time, the child's blood glucose rises higher. Levels as high as 400 to 600 mg/dl (22.2 to 33.3 mmol/L) are not uncommon, but levels as low as 300 (16.6 mmol/L) are possible. The child's blood is like thick maple syrup and doesn't circulate as freely as normal. The large amount of water leaving the body with the glucose depletes important substances such as sodium and potassium. The vomiting causes the child to lose more fluids and body substances. All these abnormalities cause the child to become very drowsy and possibly lose consciousness.

This situation is called *diabetic ketoacidosis,* and if it isn't identified and corrected quickly, the child can die.

Investigating the causes of type 1 diabetes

Type 1 diabetes is an *autoimmune disease,* meaning that your body is unkind enough to react against — and, in this case, destroy — a vital part of itself, namely the insulin-producing beta (B) cells of the pancreas.

You may wonder how doctors can know in advance that certain people will develop diabetes. The method of predicting isn't 100 percent accurate, but people who get type 1 diabetes more often have certain abnormal characteristics on their chromosomes that are not present in people who don't get diabetes. Doctors can look for these abnormal characteristics on your DNA. But having these abnormal characteristics doesn't guarantee that you'll get diabetes.

Another essential factor in predicting whether you will develop diabetes is your exposure to something in the environment, most likely a virus. I discuss this factor in detail in the next section.

Getting type 1 diabetes

To develop diabetes, most people also have to come in contact with something in the environment that triggers the destruction of their *beta cells,* the cells that make insulin. Doctors think that this environmental trigger is probably a virus, and they've identified several viruses that may be to blame. Doctors think they are the same viruses that cause the common cold.

Persons with type 1 diabetes probably get the virus just like any cold virus — from someone else who has the virus who sneezes on them. But because they also have the genetic tendency, they get type 1 diabetes.

This type of virus can cause diabetes by attacking your pancreas directly and diminishing your ability to produce insulin, which quickly creates the diabetic condition in your body. The virus can also cause diabetes if it's made up of a substance that is also naturally present in your pancreas. If the virus and your pancreas possess the same substance, the antibodies that your body produces to fight off the virus will also attack the shared substance in your pancreas, leaving you in the same condition as if the virus itself attacked your pancreas.

A small number (about 10 percent) of patients who develop type 1 diabetes don't seem to need an environmental factor to trigger the diabetes. In them, the disease is entirely an autoimmune destruction of the beta cells. If you fall into this category of people with diabetes, you may have other autoimmune diseases, such as autoimmune thyroid disease.

Preventing type 1 diabetes

Type 1 diabetes is an excellent candidate for two types of preventative treatments that should be available to patients in the not-too-distant future:

- ✔ In order to prevent diabetes, you will be able to undergo treatments before the disease starts, which is a method called *primary prevention.* Possible candidates for primary prevention are people with family histories of diabetes.

  If you fall into that category, your doctor can analyze your DNA to see whether you have the genetic material most often found in people who have diabetes. If you do, you could receive primary prevention to block the disease. An example of primary prevention for type 1 diabetes would be vaccination against the viruses that may be associated with diabetes.

- ✔ *Secondary prevention* is treatment that is given to a person with diabetes after the disease is triggered but before the person becomes sick. In order to try secondary prevention, your doctor must be able to recognize that diabetes has begun, even though you aren't sick. And months to years must pass between diagnosis and the onset of symptoms in order to have enough time for the treatment to prevent sickness.

  A lot of trials of secondary prevention are underway, though most show only partial success. The most prevalent methods of secondary prevention for type 1 diabetes attempt to block the autoimmune disease from destroying all of your pancreas's beta cells.

Examining Type 2 Diabetes

Most people with type 2 diabetes, which used to be
known as *adult onset diabetes* or *noninsulin dependent
diabetes,* are over the age of 40. Your chances of getting type 2 diabetes increase as you get older.
Because the symptoms are so mild at first, you may
not notice them. You may ignore these symptoms for
years before they become bothersome enough to con-
sult your doctor.

So type 2 diabetes is a disease of gradual onset rather
than the severe emergency that can herald type 1 diabetes. No autoimmunity is involved in type 2 diabetes, so no antibodies are found. Doctors believe that
no virus is involved in the onset of type 2 diabetes.

Recent statistics show that worldwide, ten times
more people have type 2 diabetes than type 1 diabetes. Although type 2 is the much more prevalent type
of diabetes, those with type 2 diabetes seem to have
milder severity of complications (such as eye disease
and kidney disease) from diabetes.

Identifying symptoms of type 2 diabetes

A fairly large percentage of the U.S. population
(approximately 16 to 18 million people) has type 2
diabetes. The numbers are on the rise, and one
reason is an increase in the incidence of obesity,
which is a risk factor for type 2 diabetes. If you're
obese, you are considerably more likely to acquire
type 2 diabetes than you would be if you maintained
your ideal weight.

The following signs and symptoms are good indicators that you have type 2 diabetes. If you experience two or more of these symptoms, call your doctor:

✔ **Fatigue:** Type 2 diabetes makes you tired because your body's cells aren't getting the glucose fuel that they need. Even though you have plenty of insulin in your blood, your body is resistant to its actions.

✔ **Frequent urination and thirst:** As with type 1 diabetes, you find yourself urinating more frequently than usual, which dehydrates your body and leaves you thirsty.

✔ **Blurred vision:** The lenses of your eyes swell and shrink as your blood glucose levels rise and fall. Your vision blurs because your eyes can't adjust quickly enough to these lens changes.

✔ **Slow healing of skin, gum, and urinary infections:** Your white blood cells, which help with healing and defend your body against infections, don't function correctly in the high-glucose environment present in your body when it has diabetes. Unfortunately, the bugs that cause infections thrive in the same high-glucose environment. So diabetes leaves your body especially susceptible to infections.

✔ **Genital itching:** Yeast infections also love a high-glucose environment. So diabetes is often accompanied by the itching and discomfort of yeast infections.

✔ **Numbness in the feet or legs:** You experience numbness because of a common long-term complication of diabetes called *neuropathy*. The speed with which a nervous impulse travels down a nerve fiber is called the *nerve conduction velocity*. In diabetic neuropathy, the nerve conduction velocity (NCV) is slowed.

If you notice numbness and neuropathy along with the other symptoms of diabetes, you probably have had the disease for quite a while, because neuropathy takes more than five years to develop in a diabetic environment.

✔ **Heart disease:** Heart disease occurs much more often in type 2s than in the nondiabetic population. But the heart disease may appear when you are merely glucose-intolerant (which I explain in the next section), before you actually have diagnosable diabetes.

The signs and symptoms of type 2 diabetes are similar in some cases to the symptoms of type 1 diabetes (which I cover in the "Identifying symptoms of type 1 diabetes" section, earlier in this chapter), but in many ways they are different. The following list shows some of the differences between symptoms in type 1 and type 2 diabetes:

✔ **Age of onset:** People with type 1 diabetes are usually younger than those with type 2 diabetes. However, the increasing incidence of type 2 diabetes in overweight children is making this difference less useful for separating type 1 and type 2 diabetes.

✔ **Body weight:** Those with type 1 diabetes are thin or normal in weight, but obesity is a common characteristic of people with type 2 diabetes.

✔ **Level of glucose:** People with type 1 diabetes have higher glucose levels at the onset of the disease. Those with type 1 diabetes usually have blood glucose levels of 300 to 400 mg/dl (16.6 to 22.2 mmol/L), and those with type 2 diabetes usually have blood glucose levels of 200 to 250 mg/dl (11.1 to 13.9 mmol/L).

✔ **Severity of onset:** Type 1 diabetes usually has a much more severe onset, but type 2 diabetes gradually shows its symptoms.

Investigating the causes of type 2 diabetes

If you've been diagnosed with type 2 diabetes, you're probably shocked and curious about why you developed the disease. Doctors have learned quite a bit about the causes of type 2 diabetes. For example, they know that type 2 diabetes runs in families.

Usually, people with type 2 diabetes can find a relative who has had the disease. Therefore, doctors consider type 2 diabetes to be much more of a genetic disease than type 1 diabetes. In studies of identical twins, when one twin has type 2 diabetes, the likelihood that type 2 diabetes will develop in the other twin is nearly 100 percent.

People with type 2 diabetes have plenty of insulin in their bodies (unlike people with type 1 diabetes), but their bodies respond to the insulin in abnormal ways. Those with type 2 diabetes are *insulin resistant,* meaning that their bodies resist the normal, healthy functioning of insulin. This resistance, combined with not having enough insulin to overcome the insulin resistance, causes type 2 diabetes.

Before obesity or lack of exercise (or diabetes for that matter) is present, future type 2 patients already show signs of insulin resistance. First, the amount of insulin in their blood is elevated compared to normal people. Second, a shot of insulin doesn't reduce the blood glucose in these insulin-resistant people nearly as much as it does in people without insulin resistance. (See Chapter 5 to find out more about insulin shots in diabetes.)

When your body needs to make extra insulin just to keep your blood glucose normal, your insulin is, obviously, less effective than it should be — which means that you have *impaired glucose tolerance.* Your body goes through impaired glucose tolerance before you actually have diabetes because your blood glucose is still lower than the levels needed for a diagnosis of diabetes (see Chapter 1).

When you have impaired glucose tolerance and you add other factors such as weight gain, a sedentary lifestyle, and aging, your pancreas can't keep up with your insulin demands, and you become diabetic.

Another factor that comes into play when doctors make a diagnosis of type 2 diabetes is the release of sugar from your liver, known as your *hepatic glucose output.* People with type 2 diabetes have high glucose levels in the morning after having fasted all night.

You'd think that your glucose would be low in the morning if you haven't eaten any sugar. But your liver is a storage bank for a lot of glucose, and it can make even more from other substances in the body. As your insulin resistance increases, your liver begins to release glucose inappropriately, and your fasting blood glucose level rises.

Dispelling mistaken beliefs about type 2

People often think that the following factors cause type 2 diabetes, but they actually have nothing to do with the onset of the disease:

✔ **Sugar:** Eating excessive amounts of sugar doesn't cause diabetes, but it may bring out the disease to the extent that it makes you fat. Eating too much protein or fat will do the same thing.

✔ **Emotions:** Changes in your emotions don't play a large role in the development of type 2 diabetes, but they may be very important in dealing with diabetes mellitus and subsequent control.

✔ **Stress:** Too much stress isn't a major factor that causes diabetes.

✔ **Antibodies:** Antibodies against islet cells are not a major factor in type 2 diabetes (see the section "Investigating the causes of type 1 diabetes," earlier in this chapter). Type 2 diabetes isn't an autoimmune disease like type 1.

✔ **Gender:** Males and females are equally as likely to develop type 2 diabetes. Gender doesn't play a role in the onset of this disease.

✔ **Diabetic ketoacidosis:** Type 2 diabetes isn't generally associated with diabetic ketoacidosis. People with type 2 diabetes are ketosis resistant, except under extremely severe stress caused by infections or trauma.

Getting type 2 diabetes

Genetic inheritance causes type 2 diabetes, but environmental factors such as obesity and lack of exercise trigger the disease. People with type 2 diabetes are insulin resistant before they become obese or sedentary. Aging, poor eating habits, obesity, and failure to exercise combine to bring out the disease.

Here's an interesting fact: Spouses of people with type 2 diabetes are at higher risk of developing diabetes and should be screened just like relatives of diabetics. Why? Because they share the environmental risk factors for diabetes, such as poor diet and a sedentary lifestyle.

Some early warning signs appear in the population that's most at risk to develop type 2 diabetes. People with type 2 diabetes often have a history of malnutrition at a young age. Perhaps these people didn't make enough insulin-producing cells when they were young because they didn't need them for their reduced food intake. When someone like this is presented with ample supplies of food at an older age, her pancreas may not have enough insulin-producing cells to handle the load.

Preventing type 2 diabetes

Doctors can predict type 2 diabetes years in advance of its actual diagnosis by studying the close relatives of people who have the condition. This early warning period offers plenty of time to try techniques of primary prevention (which I explain in the "Preventing type 1 diabetes" section, earlier in this chapter).

After a doctor discovers that someone's blood glucose levels are high and diagnoses type 2 diabetes, complications such as eye disease and kidney disease usually take ten or more years to develop in that person. During this time, doctors can apply secondary prevention techniques.

Because so many people suffer from type 2 diabetes, doctors have had a wealth of people to study in order to determine the most important environmental factors that turn a genetic predisposition to type 2 diabetes into a clinical disease. The following are the major environmental factors:

✔ **High body mass index:** The *body mass index (BMI)* is the way that doctors look at weight in relation to height. BMI is a better indicator of a healthy weight than just weight alone, because a person who weighs 150 pounds and is 62 inches tall is overweight, but a person who weighs 150 pounds and is 70 inches tall is thin.

You can easily determine your BMI by using the following formula: Multiply your weight (in pounds) by 705, then divide that number by your height (in inches). Divide that result by your height (in inches) again. If you use the metric system, divide your weight in kilograms by your height in meters and divide that result by your height in meters again. Using this formula, the 150-pound person with a height of 62 inches has a BMI of 27.5, while the person with the height of 70 inches has a BMI of 21.6. The result is expressed in kilograms per meter squared (kg/m^2).

Current guidelines state that a person with a BMI from 25 to 29.9 is overweight, and a person with a BMI of 30 or greater is obese. A BMI between 20 and 25 is considered normal.

✔ **Physical inactivity:** Physical inactivity has a high association with diabetes, as evidenced in many studies. Former athletes have diabetes less often than nonathletes. A study of nurses' health showed that women who were physically active on a regular basis had diabetes only two-thirds as often as the couch potatoes. A study conducted in Hawaii, which did not include any obese people, showed that the occurrence of diabetes was greatest for people who don't exercise.

✔ **Central distribution of fat:** When people with diabetes become fat, they tend to carry the extra weight as centrally distributed fat, also known as *visceral fat*. You check your visceral fat when you measure your waistline, because this type of fat stays around your midsection. So a person with visceral fat is more apple-shaped than pear-shaped. Visceral fat also happens to be the type of fat that probably comes and goes most easily on your body, and it is relatively easy to lose when you diet. Visceral fat seems to cause more insulin resistance than fat in other areas, and it is also correlated with the occurrence of coronary artery disease.

If you have a lot of visceral fat, losing just 5 to 10 percent of your weight may very dramatically reduce your chance of diabetes or a heart attack.

✔ **Low intake of dietary fiber:** Populations with a high prevalence of diabetes tend to eat a diet that is low in fiber. Dietary fiber seems to be protective against diabetes, because it slows down the rate at which glucose enters the bloodstream.

If you recognize any of the preceding factors in your body or lifestyle, you can correct them in time to prevent diabetes. Type 2 diabetes allows the high-risk individual or the diagnosed person the time to work toward prevention or control of the disease.

Understanding Gestational Diabetes

If you're pregnant (yes, this excludes you men) and you've never had diabetes before, during your pregnancy you could acquire a form of diabetes called *gestational diabetes*. If you already have diabetes when you become pregnant, that is called *pregestational diabetes*. Gestational diabetes occurs in about 2 percent of all pregnancies.

During your pregnancy, you can acquire gestational diabetes because the growing fetus and the placenta create various hormones to help the fetus grow and develop properly. Some of these hormones have other characteristics, such as anti-insulin properties, that decrease your body's sensitivity to insulin, increase glucose production, and can cause diabetes.

At approximately your 20th week of pregnancy, your body produces enough of these hormones to block your insulin's normal actions and cause diabetes. After you give birth, when the fetus and placenta are no longer in your body, their anti-insulin hormones are gone and your diabetes disappears.

Even though gestational diabetes subsides after you give birth, more than half of the women who experience gestational diabetes develop type 2 diabetes within 15 years after the pregnancy. This high likelihood of type 2 diabetes probably results from a genetic susceptibility to diabetes in these women, which is magnified by the large amount of anti-insulin hormones in their bodies during pregnancy.

Your obstetrician should do a test for gestational diabetes around the 24th to 28th week of your pregnancy.

Recognizing Other Types of Diabetes

Cases of diabetes other than type 1, type 2, or gestational are rare and usually don't cause severe diabetes in the people who have them. But occasionally one of these other types is responsible for a more severe case of diabetes, so you should know that they exist. The following sections give you a brief rundown of the symptoms and causes for other types of diabetes.

Diabetes due to loss or disease of pancreatic tissue

If you have a disease, such as cancer, that necessitates the removal of some of your pancreas, you lose your pancreas's valuable insulin-producing beta cells, and your body becomes diabetic.

This form of diabetes isn't always severe because you lose glucagon, another hormone found in your pancreas, after your pancreatic surgery. Glucagon blocks insulin action in your body, so when your body has less glucagon, it can function with less insulin, leaving you with a milder case of diabetes.

Diabetes due to iron overload

Another disease that damages the pancreas, as well as the liver, the heart, the joints, and the nervous system, is *hemochromatosis*. This condition results from excessive absorption of iron into the blood. When the blood deposits too much iron into these organs, damage can occur. This hereditary condition is present in 1 of every 200 people in the United States; half of those who have it develop a clinical disease, sometimes diabetes.

Hemochromatosis is less common in younger women, who are protected by the monthly loss of iron that occurs with menstrual bleeding. This finding has led to the current treatment for hemochromatosis, which is removing blood from the patient regularly until the blood iron returns to normal and then repeating the procedure occasionally to keep iron levels normal. If treatment is done early enough (before organs are damaged), complications, such as diabetes, are avoidable.

Diabetes due to other diseases

Your body contains a number of hormones that block insulin action or have actions that are opposed to insulin's actions. You produce these hormones in glands other than your pancreas. If you get a tumor on one of these hormone-producing glands, the gland sometimes produces excessive levels of the hormones that act in opposition to insulin. Usually, this gives you simple glucose intolerance rather than diabetes because your pancreas makes extra insulin to combat the hormones. But if you have a genetic tendency to develop diabetes, you may develop diabetes in this case.

Diabetes due to hormone treatments for other diseases

If you take hormones to treat a disease other than diabetes, those hormones could cause diabetes in your body. The hormone that is most likely to cause diabetes in this situation is *hydrocortisone,* an anti-inflammatory agent used in diseases of inflammation, such as arthritis. (Similar drugs are prednisone and dexamethasone.)

 If you take hydrocortisone and you have the symptoms of diabetes listed in earlier sections of this chapter, talk to your doctor.

Diabetes due to other drugs

If you're taking other commonly used drugs, be aware that some of them raise your blood glucose as a side effect. Some antihypertensive drugs, especially hydrochlorothiazide, raise your blood glucose level. Niacin, a drug commonly used for lowering cholesterol, also raises your blood glucose.

 If you have a genetic tendency toward diabetes, taking these drugs may be enough to give you the disease.

Chapter 3

Glucose Monitoring and Other Tests

*Y*ou're among the most fortunate people with diabetes who have ever lived. Most of the products and treatments I cover in this book weren't available just 25 years ago. And the new products coming along will knock your socks off. (But be sure to put them back on because you should not go barefoot!)

In this chapter, you discover all you need to know to put your diabetes in its proper place. You find out how well you're currently controlling your blood glucose, whether complications are beginning to show up, and what changes you need to make in your therapy to reverse or slow the progression of these complications.

Testing, Testing: Tests You Need to Stay Healthy

 Certain procedures should be done by your doctor (and you, if feasible) according to the following schedule:

- ✔ Evaluate your blood glucose measurements at each visit.
- ✔ Obtain hemoglobin A1c four times a year if you take insulin and twice a year if you don't.
- ✔ Check for microalbuminuria once a year.
- ✔ Have a dilated eye examination by an ophthal-mologist once a year.
- ✔ Examine your bare feet at each visit.
- ✔ Have an ankle-brachial index performed at least every five years.
- ✔ Obtain a lipid panel once a year.
- ✔ Measure your blood pressure at each visit.
- ✔ Measure your weight at each visit.

I discuss each of these tests in the sections that follow. These tests are the minimum standards for proper care of diabetes. If an abnormality is found, the frequency of testing increases to check on the response to treatment.

Monitoring Blood Glucose: It's a Must

Insulin was extracted and used for the first time more than 80 years ago. Since that time, nothing has improved the life of the person with diabetes as much as the ability to measure his or her own blood glucose with a drop of blood.

Basically, two kinds of test strips are used today. Both require that glucose in a drop of your blood reacts with an enzyme. In one strip, the reaction produces a color. A meter then reads the amount of color to give a glucose reading. In the other strip, the reaction produces electrons, and a meter converts the amount of electrons into a glucose reading.

A person who works hard to control his glucose, can experience tremendous variation in glucose levels in a relatively short time. This is especially true in association with food, but variations can occur even in the fasting state before breakfast. This is why multiple tests are needed.

How often should you test?

How often you test is determined by the kind of diabetes you have, the kind of treatment you're using, and the level of stability of your blood glucose.

✔ **If you have type 1 or type 2 diabetes and you're taking insulin, you need to test before each meal and at bedtime.** The reason is that you're constantly using this information to make adjustments in your insulin dose. No matter how good you think your control is, you cannot feel the level of the blood glucose without testing unless you're hypoglycemic.

People with type 1 diabetes should occasionally test one hour after a meal and in the middle of the night to see just how high their glucose goes after eating and whether it drops too low in the middle of the night. These results guide you and your physician to make the changes you need.

✔ **If you have type 2 diabetes and you're on pills or just diet and exercise, you need to test before breakfast and dinner.** I'm assuming that you're fairly stable as shown by mostly good blood glucose tests (in the range of 80 to 120 mg/dl) and by the hemoglobin A1c (which I discuss later in this chapter).

I even have some of my most stable patients testing only once a day, alternating a prebreakfast test with a presupper test on consecutive days. Any less testing than that is not enough to keep you aware of the state of your control.

The blood glucose test can be useful many other times of day:

✔ If you eat something off your diet and want to test its effect on your glucose, do a test.

✔ If you're about to exercise, a blood glucose test can tell you whether you need to eat before starting the exercise or can use the exercise to bring your glucose down.

✔ If your diabetes is temporarily unstable and you're about to drive, you may want to test before getting into the car to make sure that you're not on the verge of hypoglycemia.

You're not being graded on your glucose test results. The human body has too much variation in it to expect that each time you take the same medication, do the same exercise, eat the same way, and feel the same emotionally, you'll get the same test result.

Keep in mind that the occasional blood glucose test done in your doctor's office is of little or no value in understanding the big picture of your glucose control. It's like trying to visualize an entire painting by Seurat (who painted using dots of color) by looking at one dot on the canvas.

How do you perform the test?

If you don't already own a blood glucose meter, be sure to check out the next section. All meters require a drop of blood, usually from the finger. You place the blood on a specific part of a test strip and allow enough time, usually between five seconds and one minute, for a reaction to occur. Some strips allow you to add more blood within 30 seconds if the quantity is insufficient. In less than a minute, the meter reads the product of that reaction, which is determined by the amount of glucose in the blood sample.

Keep the following tips in mind when you're testing your glucose:

✔ If you have trouble getting blood, you can use a rubber band at the point where your finger joins your hand. You'll be amazed at the flow of blood.

✔ Testing blood from sites other than your fingers is generally reliable, except for an hour after eating or immediately after exercise.

✔ Some meters use whole blood, and some use the liquid part of the blood, called the *plasma.* A lab glucose tests the plasma. The whole blood value is about 12 percent less than the plasma value, so it is important to know which you're measuring. The various recommendations for appropriate levels of glucose are plasma values unless specifically stated otherwise. Most of the newer meters are calibrated to give a plasma reading, but check yours to be sure.

✔ Studies have shown that the qualities of test strips, which are loose in a vial, deteriorate rapidly if the vial is left open. Be sure to cap the vial. Two hours of exposure to air may ruin the strips. Strips that are individually foil-wrapped do not have this problem.

✔ Do not let others use your meter. Their test results will be mixed in with your tests when they are downloaded into a computer. In addition, a meter invariably gets a little blood on it and can be a source of infection.

Choosing a Blood Glucose Meter

So many meters are on the market that you may be confused about which one to use. One consideration that should play little part in your decision is the cost of the meter. Most manufacturers are happy to practically give you the meter so that you're forced to buy their test strips. Each manufacturer makes a different test strip, and they're not interchangeable in other machines. Some even make a different strip for each different machine that they make.

Because the meters are so cheap and the science is changing so rapidly, you should get a new meter every year or two to make sure that you have state-of-the-art equipment. The cost of test strips is generally about the same from meter to meter, so the cost of strips doesn't have to play a big role in your meter decision.

Your doctor may have a meter that he or she prefers to work with because a computer program can download the test results from the meter and display them in a certain way. This analysis can be enormously helpful in deciding how to alter your therapy for the best control of your glucose.

Any meter you buy should have a memory that records the time and date so you can read that information along with the glucose result. The memory should handle at least 100 glucose values if you test four times a day; 100 values represents 25 days at this testing frequency.

Don't buy a meter without the capability to download the results to a data management system in a computer. Bring your meter with you to your appointments so that your doctor can download your glucose test results and evaluate them with the aid of a data management system. Evaluating pages of glucose readings in a log book is virtually impossible.

Your insurance company also may mandate a certain meter, in which case you may have no choice.

Tracking Your Glucose over Time: Hemoglobin A1c

Individual blood glucose tests are great for deciding how you're doing at that moment and what to do to make it better, but they don't give the big picture. They are just a moment in time. Glucose can change a great deal even in an hour. What you need is a test that gives an integrated picture of many days, weeks, or even months of blood glucose levels. The test that accomplishes this important task is called the *hemoglobin A1c*.

With this test, you can look back and say that you were or were not in control of your blood glucose for whatever period of time the test reviews. This is a perfect test, for example, for the diabetic woman who wants to get pregnant. She can know whether her blood glucose has been well controlled before she tries to conceive. If it has not, she can wait until the test shows good control before getting pregnant.

Unfortunately, all labs do not do the hemoglobin A1c test the same way. You need to know the normal value in the lab where you do the test. Fortunately, each lab usually has a column on its result form showing the normal values for each test. Still, this situation can create confusion.

The standard method should be the way it was done in the Diabetes Control and Complications Trial, the study that showed that controlling the blood glucose prevents complications in type 1 diabetes. In that study, a normal level was about 6.05 percent. Figure 3-1 shows you the correlation between the hemoglobin A1c and the blood glucose when this method is used.

As you can see in the figure, a normal hemoglobin A1c of less than 6 percent corresponds to a blood glucose of less than 120, while a fair hemoglobin A1c of 7 percent reflects an average blood glucose of 150.

Large-scale studies have shown that the average hemoglobin A1c in the United States for type 2 diabetes is around 9.4 percent, which means the average blood glucose is 220. The American Diabetes Association recommends taking action to control the blood glucose if the hemoglobin A1c is 8 percent or greater, with the goal being less than 7 percent.

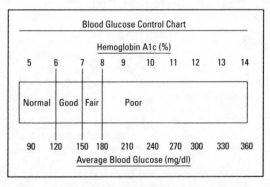

Figure 3-1: Comparison between hemoglobin A1c and blood glucose.

Your physician should test for hemoglobin A1c as follows:

- ✔ Four times a year if you have type 1 or type 2 diabetes and are on insulin
- ✔ Two times a year if you have type 2 diabetes and are not on insulin

Bayer Health Care has a clever home version of the hemoglobin A1c, called *A1c Now*. You do a finger stick to produce a large drop of blood. The blood is mixed with a solution that is provided, and a sample of that mixture is placed in the testing device. Eight minutes later, the hemoglobin A1c appears in the device window. The device is then discarded. The device appears to be highly accurate and may save the trouble of going to a lab for this test.

Another option is to collect your own blood specimen and send it to a company that will run the test and give you and your doctor a result. The companies currently doing this include

- ✔ AccuBase A1c Glycohemoglobin (www.diabetes technologies.com)
- ✔ Appraise A1c Diabetes Monitoring System (www.matria.com)
- ✔ A1c at Home (www.flexsite.com)
- ✔ BioSafe A1c Hemoglobin Test Kit (www.ebio safe.com)
- ✔ SimpleChoice A1c (www.spectrx.com)

Testing for Kidney Damage: Microalbuminuria

The finding of very small but abnormal amounts of protein in the urine, called *microalbuminuria,* is the earliest sign that high glucose may be damaging your kidneys. When microalbuminuria is found, you still have time to reverse any damage.

 As soon as you are diagnosed with type 2 diabetes, and within five years of being diagnosed with type 1, your doctor must order a urine test for microalbuminuria. If the test is negative, it must be repeated annually. If the test is positive, it should be done a second time to verify the result. If the second test is positive, your doctor should do the following:

✔ **Put you on a drug called an ACE inhibitor.** After you have been on this drug for some months, the test for microalbuminuria can be repeated to see whether it has turned negative. The ACE inhibitor can be stopped and restarted later if microalbuminuria appears again.

✔ **Bring your blood glucose under the tightest control possible.** This helps to reverse the damaging process as well.

✔ **Normalize your body fats so that your cholesterol and triglycerides are made normal.** Elevated cholesterol and triglycerides have been found to damage the kidneys. (See the section "Tracking Cholesterol and Other Fats," later in this chapter.)

 Doing this simple little test can protect your kidneys from damage. Ask your doctor about it if you think it has never been done. Show him or her this book if the doctor is unclear as to why it's performed.

Checking for Eye Problems

All people with diabetes need to have a dilated eye exam done annually by an ophthalmologist or optometrist. No other physician, including the endocrinologist (yours truly excepted, of course), can do the exam properly.

For this exam, the doctor instills drops into your eyes and uses various instruments to examine the pressure, the appearance of your lens, and, most importantly, the retina of your eye. All kinds of treatments can be done if abnormalities are found, but they must be discovered first.

 This test is something you must demand. Your doctor must refer you to an ophthalmologist or optometrist every year. Better yet, set up the appointment yourself with the eye doctor's nurse at the end of your first visit so that you are reminded about it each year.

Examining Your Feet

Unfortunately, foot problems often end in amputation. An amputation is really evidence of inadequate care. The doctor isn't necessarily at fault here. The doctor sees you once in a while. You're with yourself much more often.

 If you have any problem sensing touch with your feet, you need to take the following precautions:

✔ Use your eyes to examine your feet every day.

✔ Use your hand to test hot water before you step into it so that you do not get burned.

✔ Shake out your shoes before you step into them to make sure no stone or other object is inside them.

- ✔ Do not go barefoot.
- ✔ Keep the skin of your feet moist by soaking them in water, drying them, and applying a moisturizing lotion.

 Your doctor can test your ability to feel an injury by using a 10-gram filament, but, again, that is done only when you have an appointment. You can obtain one of these filaments for yourself. Call the National Diabetes Information Clearinghouse at 800-438-5383 and ask for the "Feet Can Last a Lifetime" package. Better yet, go to http://ndep. nih.gov/media/Feet_HCGuide.pdf to learn how to protect your feet and how to get the kit.

The other part of a foot examination involves checking the circulation of blood to your feet. To accomplish this, your doctor does a measurement called an *ankle-bra-chial index* at least once every five years. The systolic blood pressure is measured in the ankle and the arm.

The value for the ankle is divided by the value for the arm. An index of greater than 0.9 is considered normal. A value between 0.4 and 0.9 indicates peripheral vascular disease, while a value less than 0.4 indicates severe disease.

The ankle-brachial index should be done for any diabetic over age 50. Patients under 50 require the study if risk factors such as smoking, high cholesterol, and high blood pressure are present.

Tracking Cholesterol and Other Fats

Most people these days know the level of their total cholesterol, but other tests that show levels of various types of fats in the blood are needed are well.

Cholesterol is a type of fat that circulates in the blood in small packages called *lipoproteins.* These tiny round particles contain fat (*lipo,* as in liposuction) and protein. Because cholesterol doesn't dissolve in water, it would separate from the blood if it weren't surrounded by the protein, just like oil separates from water in salad dressing.

A second kind of fat found in the lipoproteins is *triglyceride.* Triglyceride actually represents the form of most of the fat you eat each day. Although you may eat only a gram or less of cholesterol (an egg yolk has one-third of a gram of cholesterol), you eat up to 100 grams of triglyceride a day. The fat in animal meats is mostly triglycerides.

You don't have to fast to do a test for total cholesterol and HDL cholesterol. However, you do need to fast for eight hours to find out your LDL cholesterol, because the blood has to be cleared of chylomicrons, which rise greatly when you eat.

 You should have a *fasting lipid panel* at least once each year. That means no food after supper the night before. A fasting lipid panel gives you your total cholesterol, your LDL cholesterol, your HDL cholesterol, and your triglyceride levels.

The current recommendations for the levels of these fats in terms of the risk for coronary artery disease are as follows:

- **✔ LDL Cholesterol**

    Higher risk: Greater than 130

    Borderline: 100 to 129

    Lower risk: Less than 100

- **✔ HDL Cholesterol**

    Higher risk: Less than 35

    Borderline: 35 to 45

Lower risk: Greater than 45

✔ **Triglycerides**

Higher risk: Greater than 400

Borderline: 200 to 399

Lower risk: Less than 200

The risk goes up as the LDL cholesterol goes up and the HDL cholesterol goes down. A huge study of thousands of citizens of Framingham, Massachusetts, shows that you can get a good picture of the risk by dividing the total cholesterol by the HDL cholesterol. If this result is less than 4.5, the risk is lower. If it's greater than 4.5, you're at higher risk for coronary artery disease. The higher it is, the worse the risk.

Diabetes adds its own complication because of the metabolic syndrome. In the metabolic syndrome, the total cholesterol may not be very high, but the HDL cholesterol is low and the triglycerides are elevated. These patients also have a lot of a dangerous form of LDL cholesterol, so they are at higher risk for coronary artery disease. This increased risk must be taken into account in considering treatment for the fats.

In deciding whether and how to treat the fats, you have to consider other risk factors for coronary artery disease. You're at highest risk if you already have coronary artery disease, stroke, or peripheral vascular disease. You're at high risk if you

✔ Are a male over 45

✔ Are a female over 55

✔ Smoke cigarettes

✔ Have high blood pressure

✔ Have HDL cholesterol less than 35

✔ Have a father or brother who had a heart attack before age 55

✔ Have a mother or sister who had a heart attack before age 65

✔ Have a body mass index greater than 30

The treatment for abnormal fats then depends on your risk category and level of LDL cholesterol (see Table 3-1).

Table 3-1	Your Treatment Based on Risk Category	
Risk	**Dietary Treatment If LDL Greater Than**	**Diet and Drug Treatment If LDL Greater Than**
Low	100	100
High	130	160
Very high	160	190

All these decisions depend on obtaining a lipid (fat) panel.

Measuring Blood Pressure

People with diabetes have high blood pressure more often than the nondiabetic population for a lot of reasons:

✔ People with diabetes get kidney disease.

✔ People with diabetes have increased sensitivity to salt, which raises blood pressure.

✔ People with diabetes lack the nighttime fall in blood pressure that normally occurs in people without diabetes.

Doctors generally agree that a normal blood pressure is less than 140/90. For years, the *diastolic blood pressure* (the lower reading) was considered more damaging, and an elevation in that pressure was treated with greater importance than an elevation in the *systolic blood pressure* (the higher reading). Recent studies have shown that the systolic blood pressure, not the diastolic blood pressure, may be more important.

All the complications of diabetes are made worse by an elevation in blood pressure, especially diabetic kidney disease but also eye disease, heart disease, nerve disease, peripheral vascular disease, and cerebral arterial disease.

The most recent evidence of the importance of controlling blood pressure in diabetes comes from the United Kingdom Prospective Diabetes Study, published in late 1998. This study found that a lowering of blood pressure by 10 mm systolic and 5 mm diastolic resulted in a 24 percent reduction in any diabetic complication and a 32 percent reduction in death related to diabetes.

Controlling the blood pressure is absolutely essential in diabetes. The goal in diabetes is an even lower blood pressure than in the nondiabetic because studies have shown that lower normal blood pressures result in less diabetic damage than higher normal blood pressures. Your blood pressure should be no higher than 130/80.

Your doctor should measure blood pressure at every visit. Better yet, get a blood pressure device and measure it yourself. If you detect an elevation, bring it to the attention of your doctor.

For much more information on every aspect of high blood pressure, see my book *High Blood Pressure For Dummies* (Wiley).

Checking Your Weight and BMI

Body Mass Index (BMI) is a measurement that relates weight to height. A tall person has a lower BMI than a short person of the same weight. (See Chapter 2 for more on BMI, including instructions for calculating your own BMI.) A person with a BMI under 20 is considered slim. A person with a BMI from 20 to 25 is normal. A person with a BMI from 25 to 29.9 is overweight, and a person with a BMI over 30 is obese. By this definition, more than half the people in the United States are overweight or obese.

You cannot step on a scale and get a reading of your BMI, but you can get your weight. This is one of the easiest measurements in medicine. Your doctor should measure your weight at every visit.

Maintaining a BMI in the normal range makes controlling your diabetes and blood pressure easier. Also, you must eliminate obesity as a risk factor for coronary artery disease.

Testing for Ketones

When your blood glucose rises above 250 mg/dl (13.9 mmol/L), or if you are pregnant with diabetes and your blood glucose is below 60 mg/dl (3.3 mmol/L), it's a good idea to check for *ketones* — products of the breakdown of fats. Finding ketones means that your body has turned to fat for energy. If you have high glucose and find ketones, you may need more insulin. If you have low glucose and find ketones during pregnancy, you may need more carbohydrates in your diet.

Testing for ketones is done by inserting a test strip into your urine and observing a purple color. The deeper the color, the greater the ketone level. If you find a large amount of ketones, you should contact your physician.

Testing the C-reactive Protein

C-reactive protein (CRP) is a substance in the blood that is produced by the liver when there is infection or inflammation. It can be measured with a simple blood test. Diabetes is associated with several features that suggest that inflammation plays an important role in the disease. People who develop diabetes have higher C-reactive protein than those who don't. (Other substances associated with inflammation are also elevated in diabetes.)

Drugs that improve diabetes lower the amount of C-reactive protein, which is also considered a marker for coronary artery disease.

Have your C-reactive protein measured with other blood tests about once a year. If the level is elevated, it may serve as a predictor of future diabetes or coronary artery disease. About 90 percent of healthy individuals have CRP levels less than 3, and 99 percent have levels less than 10.

Chapter 4

Investigating Oral Medications

*F*or years, insulin shots (see Chapter 5) were the only treatment available for diabetes. Most people do not care for shots. You may be an exception, but I doubt it. Fortunately, drugs that can be taken by mouth have been available for some time. One thing you should know about these pills: You can take them or leave them, but they work much better if you take them.

You should never take a drug, or a combination of drugs, as a convenient way of avoiding the basic diet and exercise that are the keys to diabetic control. (See Chapters 6 and 7 for more information on these crucial points.)

Introducing Sulfonylureas

Scientists discovered sulfonylureas accidentally when they noticed that soldiers who were given certain sulfur-containing antibiotics developed symptoms of low blood glucose. When scientists began to search for the most potent examples of this effect, they came up with several different versions of this drug. Sulfonylureas all have the following characteristics:

- ✔ They work by making the pancreas release more insulin.

- ✔ They are not effective in type 1 diabetes where the pancreas is not capable of releasing any insulin.

- ✔ Sometimes they don't work when first given (primary failure), but almost always they stop working within a few years after you start them (secondary failure). Sulfonylureas continue to be used because, for most people, they improve glucose control for at least those first few years.

- ✔ They are all capable of causing hypoglycemia.

- ✔ When you use any of a class of antibiotics called *sulfonamides,* the glucose-lowering action of the sulfonylureas is prolonged.

- ✔ They should not be taken by a pregnant woman or a nursing mother.

- ✔ They can be fairly potent when given in combination with one of the other classes of oral agents.

The original sulfonylureas from the 1950s, the first-generation sulfonylureas, are not used as initial treatment as much anymore but are actually just as useful as the newer, second-generation sulfonylureas. The old ones are just as effective, but more milligrams are required for the same effect. All the first-generation drugs are available in a generic form, which makes them less expensive. The first-generation sulfonyl-ureas include

- ✔ **Tolbutamide,** brand name Orinase. This is the only short-acting sulfonylurea. Because it is rapidly broken down in the liver, tolbutamide begins to work in one hour and is gone from the body in ten hours. It is available in 250 and 500 mg strength. Tolbutamide is usually given before each meal, but some patients require only one or two doses a day. Because it lasts for such a short time, tolbutamide is much safer in elderly people. The maximal dose is 3 grams daily (six 500 mg pills).

- ✔ **Tolazamide,** brand name Tolinase. This agent is absorbed more slowly than other sulfonylureas, so it takes 4 or more hours to notice its effects, and its activity lasts up to 20 hours. Tolazamide is available in 100, 250, and 500 mg. When more than 500 mg is needed, the dose is divided. The maximum dose is 1,000 mg. This drug is changed in the liver, but the new products produced by this change have the ability to lower the blood glucose just like tolazamide. Because the new products are then disposed of in the urine, a person with kidney disease should be careful about taking this medication.

- ✔ **Acetohexamide,** brand name Dymelor. Acetohexamide begins to work about 1 hour after it's taken and lasts for 12 hours. It comes in 250 and 500 mg strength. Acetohexamide is given in one or two doses daily, and the maximum useful dose is 1.5 grams (three 500 mg tablets). Acetohexamide is inactivated and excreted just like tolazamide, so it requires the same precautions about kidney problems.

✔ **Chlorpropamide,** brand names Diabinase and Glucamide. Chlorpropamide is the longest acting of the first-generation sulfonylureas and was responsible for many cases of hypoglycemia in the past. It is active for 24 hours or longer. Chlorpropamide causes a very prolonged hypoglycemia that sometimes requires treatment with intravenous glucose for several days. It comes in 100 and 250 mg sizes. The maximum recommended dose is 750 mg. It is broken down into other chemicals, which are also active and are slowly eliminated in the urine, so any kidney problem will greatly lengthen its time of activity. This drug is taken only once a day because it lasts so long.

Too often, doctors today do not try the first-generation drugs and go right to the second-generation pills. For many people, the second-generation pills are too potent, and hypoglycemia becomes a problem. For others, the second-generation drugs provide no greater benefit than the earlier ones. All these drugs — both first- and second-generation — suffer from the fact that, sooner or later, they no longer control the blood glucose.

Three second-generation sulfonylureas now exist:

✔ **Glyburide,** brand names Micronase, Diabeta, and Glynase. Glyburide comes in 1.25, 2.5, and 5 mg strengths. The usual starting dose is 2.5 to 5 mg with breakfast, and the maintenance dose is 1.25 to 20 mg. Glyburide leaves the body equally in the bowel movement and the urine, so patients with either liver or kidney disease are at greater risk for low blood glucose. Glyburide is carried around the bloodstream bound to proteins, so if other drugs that bind to proteins are taken, such as aspirin, the activity of glyburide may increase. When these drugs are withdrawn, the activity of glyburide may decrease. Other than hypoglycemia, the incidence of negative effects is very low.

✔ **Glipizide,** brand names Glucotrol and Glucotrol XL. Glipizide is similar to glyburide but slightly less potent so that it comes as 5 and 10 mg pills. You take it 30 minutes before food. The starting dose is 5 mg. Up to 40 mg can be given daily in several doses. Because it's less potent, glipizide is preferred in the elderly.

Glucotrol XL is an extended-release form of glipizide that lasts for 24 hours, so it usually is given as 5 or 10 mg once a day.

✔ **Glimepiride,** brand name Amaryl. This drug also lasts a longer time and is fairly potent, so it is given once a day. It comes in 1, 2, and 4 mg sizes with a maximum daily dose of 8 mg.

Meeting Metformin

Metformin, brand name Glucophage, is an entirely different kind of glucose-lowering medication. It has the following characteristics:

✔ It lowers the blood glucose mainly by reducing the production of glucose from the liver (the *hepatic* glucose output).

✔ It works for both type 1 and type 2 diabetes, because (unlike the sulfonylureas) it does not depend on stimulating insulin to work.

✔ Used by itself *(monotherapy),* it does not cause hypoglycemia.

✔ It may increase the sensitivity of the muscle cells to insulin and slow the uptake of glucose from the intestine.

- ✔ It must be taken with food because it causes gastrointestinal irritation, but this side effect declines with time.

- ✔ It's available in 500 mg, 850 mg, and 1,000 mg tablets.

- ✔ The maximum dose is 2,500 mg taken in divided doses with each meal.

- ✔ It's often associated with weight loss, possibly from the gastrointestinal irritation or because of a loss of taste for food.

- ✔ It's not recommended when you have significant liver disease, kidney disease, or heart failure.

- ✔ It's usually stopped for a day or two before surgery or an x-ray study using a dye.

- ✔ It's not recommended for use in alcoholics.

- ✔ It's not recommended for use in pregnancy or by a nursing mother.

- ✔ When given in combination with the sulfonylureas, hypoglycemia can occur. If low blood glucose is persistent, the dose of sulfonylurea is reduced.

Metformin can be a very useful drug, especially when *fasting hyperglycemia* (high blood glucose upon awakening) is present. Metformin has some positive effects on the blood fats, causing a decrease in triglycerides and LDL cholesterol and an increase in HDL cholesterol. About 10 percent of patients fail to respond to it when it is first used, and the secondary failure rate is 5 to 10 percent a year. It occasionally causes a decrease in the absorption of vitamin B_{12}, a vitamin that is important for the blood and the nervous system.

Considering Alpha-glucosidase Inhibitors

These are drugs that block the action of an enzyme in the intestine that breaks down complex carbohydrates into simple sugars that can be absorbed. Taking alpha-glucosidase inhibitors results in a slowing of the rise in glucose after meals. The carbohydrates are eventually broken down by bacteria lower down in the intestine, producing a lot of gas, abdominal pain, and diarrhea — the main drawbacks of these drugs.

Two alpha-glucosidase inhibitors currently being used are Miglitol, brand name Glyset, and Acarbose, brand name Precose. The main characteristics of these drugs are

- They're supplied in 25, 50, and 100 mg strengths.

- The recommended starting dose is 25 mg at the beginning of each meal. This dose can be increased to 50 or 100 mg three times daily, depending on the blood glucose. The highest dose is not given unless the patient weighs more than 130 pounds.

- They do not require insulin for their activity, so they work for both type 1 and type 2 diabetes.

- They do not cause hypoglycemia when used alone but do in combination with sulfonylureas. If hypoglycemia is persistent, the dose of sulfonylurea is decreased.

- They should not be used by people with intestinal disease.

- Many people do not like them because of the gastrointestinal effects.

- The lowering of glucose and hemoglobin A1c is modest at most.

Because these drugs block the breakdown of complex carbohydrates, hypoglycemia occurring with acarbose or miglitol and sulfonylurea combinations must be treated with a preparation of glucose, not more complex carbohydrates.

In my own practice, I haven't found a use for either drug. I tried acarbose on a number of patients, and even though they started at a low dose and gradually built up to a more effective level, they complained about the gas and abdominal pain and asked me to take them off the drug. Because I was not seeing much change in the blood glucose, I did not object. I see no reason to expect that miglitol would be any different.

Introducing Thiazolidinediones

This is the first group of drugs for diabetes that directly reverses insulin resistance.

Rosiglitazone

Rosiglitazone is marketed by Glaxo SmithKline as Avandia. The characteristics of rosiglitazone are

- ✔ It's available as 2, 4, and 8 mg tablets.

- ✔ Tablets are taken with or without food once a day.

- ✔ The recommended starting dose is 4 mg, and 8 mg is the maximum recommended dose. Increases in the dose are made no more often than every two to four weeks. Rosiglitazone may take three months or longer to have its maximum effect.

- ✔ Because it improves insulin resistance, this drug has its greatest effect on the blood glucose after eating, rather than the first morning glucose.

- ✔ By itself, rosiglitazone does not cause hypoglycemia. It results in hypoglycemia only when combined with insulin or sulfonylurea.

- ✔ If rosiglitazone is given to a patient on sulfonylurea or metformin, those drugs must not be stopped when the rosiglitazone is started because it takes so long for the rosiglitazone to begin to work.

- ✔ Rosiglitazone is *insulin-sparing,* meaning the body does not have to make as much insulin to control blood glucose when this drug is given.

- ✔ The drug is eliminated from the body almost entirely through the bowels, so no adjustment of the dose is needed when the kidneys are poorly functioning.

However, rosiglitazone does have some problems:

- ✔ Although rosiglitazone has not been shown to cause severe liver damage, the FDA requires that liver testing be done before starting treatment, every two months for the first year, and periodically thereafter. If the specific liver test called ALT rises more than three times the upper limit of normal, the drug must be stopped. So far, I have had no such problem after treating several hundred patients with this drug.

- ✔ Rosiglitazone causes water retention and swelling of the ankles, especially in the older population, which some people do not find tolerable. Occasionally the drug is stopped for this reason. This water retention may also be responsible for a mild decrease in red blood cells called *anemia.* The drug should not be used in people with heart failure.

- ✔ It should not be taken during pregnancy or by a nursing mother.

Rosiglitazone has been associated with an increased incidence of heart attacks. *I do not recommend it.* I have switched all my patients on rosiglitazone to pioglitazone or other drugs.

Pioglitazone

Pioglitazone, brand name Actos, has the same properties as rosiglitazone with the following differences:

- ✔ The initial dose is 15 mg once a day with or without food, but most patients require 30 or even 45 mg. It comes in all three sizes.

- ✔ In addition to restoring fertility in some women who are infertile due to insulin resistance, pioglitazone reduces estrogen levels in women taking estrogen and may result in making hormone-based contraception, such as the Pill or Depo-Provera, less effective.

- ✔ Pioglitazone has been shown to reduce bad (LDL) cholesterol particles in people with or without diabetes (as reported in *Diabetes Care,* September 2003).

- ✔ Pioglitazone has been shown to be associated with increased osteoporosis in women.

- ✔ Pioglitazone has not been shown to be associated with an increased incidence of heart attacks.

- ✔ It is authorized for use alone, with insulin, with metformin, or with a sulfonylurea.

Pioglitazone 30 mg has been combined with glimepiride 2 mg or 4 mg in a pill called Duetact by Takeda.

Presenting the Meglitinides

Each of these drugs, although they are chemically
somewhat different, has about the same activity. They
are chemically unrelated to the sulfonylureas but work
by squeezing more insulin out of the pancreas just like
the sulfonylureas do. They are taken just before meals
to stimulate insulin for only that meal.

Repaglinide

Repaglinide, brand name Prandin, was the first megli-
tinide. The characteristics of repaglinide include

- It is available as 0.5, 1, and 2 mg tablets and is
  taken up to 30 minutes before meals.

- The starting dose is 0.5 mg with a mild elevation
  of blood glucose or 1 or 2 mg if the initial blood
  glucose is higher. The dose may be doubled
  once a week to a maximum of 4 mg before
  meals.

- Because it acts through insulin, repaglinide can
  cause hypoglycemia.

- It's not recommended in pregnancy or for nursing mothers.

- It's not used with the sulfonylureas but can be
  combined with metformin. Use in combination
  with rosiglitazone has not been studied.

- Repaglinide lowers the blood glucose and the
  hemoglobin A1c effectively when used in combination with metformin.

- It's mostly broken down in the liver and leaves
  the body in the bowel movement. Therefore, if
  liver disease is present, the dose has to be
  adjusted downward.

✔ Despite the lack of excretion through the kidneys, increases in the dose have to be made more carefully when kidney impairment is present.

Experience with repaglinide has shown that it causes no problems when given with nondiabetes medications. It's bound to protein in the blood, so medications like aspirin (which also bind to protein) may, theoretically, increase its activity, but I haven't seen this as a problem with my patients.

Nateglinide

Nateglinide, brand name Starlix, is very similar to repaglinide in its activity. However, it comes in 60 and 120 mg sizes. The starting dose is usually 120 mg before each meal; if a meal is skipped, no dose is taken. If hypoglycemia occurs, the dose is lowered to 60 mg. The features of repaglinide also apply to nateglinide, other than the dosage.

DPP-4 inhibitors

This new class of drugs has a different mechanism from any of the previous classes of oral agents. There is a hormone called glucagon-like peptide-1 (GLP-1), which is made in the small intestine and has a number of positive effects for people with diabetes:

✔ It slows the movement of food in the intestine.

✔ It reduces the production of glucagon from the pancreas. Glucagon raises the blood glucose.

✔ It increases insulin levels.

✔ It decreases food intake leading to weight loss.

✔ It normalizes the blood glucose in many patients.

The only problem with GLP-1 is that it is rapidly broken down by an enzyme called DPP-4. Therefore, under usual circumstances, GLP-1 is not around long enough to have these effects in a major way.

This class of drugs, called DPP-4 inhibitors, blocks the rapid breakdown of GLP-1 and prolongs its actions. There are currently two DPP-4 inhibitors, only one of which is available for patients:

✔ **Sitagliptin:** This drug has the brand name Januvia, is made by Merck, and comes in 25 mg, 50 mg, and 100 mg. The dose is 100 mg daily. Since it is excreted by the kidneys, people with kidney disease must take lower doses. It can cause stomach discomfort.

   The problem with sitagliptin is that the amount of lowering of the hemoglobin A1c is less than 1 percent. In addition, it doesn't result in weight loss, which, I believe is the major advantage of GLP-1. Finally, it has been tested in only a few thousand patients. We don't know what unexpected side effects will show themselves after millions of people have started to use it. Therefore, I'm using it sparingly if at all in my practice until we know more about it, particularly because it doesn't have a major effect on blood glucose.

✔ **Vidagliptin:** This drug, with the brand name Galvus and made by Novartis, is very similar in its effects to sitagliptin. It has not yet been authorized for sale by the FDA.

New injectable drugs

DPP-4 inhibitors work by blocking the breakdown of the natural hormone GLP-1. Amylin Pharmaceuticals and Eli Lilly have been able to extract a substance from the venom of a lizard called the Gila Monster that acts like GLP-1 but doesn't break down nearly as fast; they call it enenatide. They've also been able to produce a second injectable substance called pramlintide with many similar properties.

Exenatide

Exenatide, which the companies call Byetta, is a powerful form of GLP-1 that lasts for several hours. It's taken within an hour before breakfast and supper. It may only be used in type 2 diabetes and comes in vials containing either 5 or 10 micrograms per dose. It may be used with metformin, a sulfonylurea or pioglitazone or combinations of those drugs. It can sometimes cause substantial weight loss and eliminate the need for all those drugs. Exenatide is associated with nausea and, rarely, can't be used because the nausea is so severe. Hypoglycemia is frequent when it is used with a sulfonylurea. At present, it is not supposed to be used with insulin.

A long-acting version of Byetta is soon to be available. It will require taking only one shot a week. Studies have shown that it controls glucose even better than twice-daily Byetta.

This drug has proved to be very valuable in the treatment of type 2 diabetes. It is sometimes necessary to use more than the maximum recommended dose of 20 micrograms a day.

Pramlintide

Pramlintide (brand name Symlin) is an extract from the same beta cells of the pancreas that produce insulin. It has a number of valuable properties for type 1 and type 2 diabetes:

  ✔ It blocks the secretion of glucagon, a major hormone that tends to raise blood glucose (see Chapter 2 for details).

✔ It slows the emptying of the stomach so that glucose is absorbed more slowly.

✔ It causes loss of appetite and weight loss.

Amylin, therefore, has an important effect on the rate at which glucose appears in the blood after eating. These effects occur when amylin reaches certain centers in the brain.

Because amylin comes from the same cells that make insulin, it's absent in type 1 diabetes just as insulin is absent in type 1 diabetes. It was thought that providing amylin to a patient with T1DM may improve the blood glucose. However, naturally occurring amylin has chemical properties that make it unusable as a pill or an injection. Mainly, it couldn't be made to dissolve in any liquid. A small change in the chemical structure made it possible to dissolve the new chemical while retaining all the properties of amylin.

Pramlintide is taken before meals that contain at least 30 grams of carbohydrate or 250 kilocalories. It does not mix with insulin. Since pramlintide is so potent, the insulin dose must be reduced by half. It can cause nausea and hypoglycemia.

The starting dose of pramlintide is 15 micrograms before meals; this is increased by 15 micrograms every three days. The maximum daily total dose is 120 micrograms.

Pramlintide has not been studied in pregnancy and while breast feeding, so it should not be used for these conditions. Children may use it.

You should probably not use pramlintide if you have hypoglycemia unawareness (see Chapter 4) or a form of diabetic neuropathy called gastro-paresis (see Chapter 5), which makes the stomach empty slowly.

Using Other Medications

Most of this chapter is devoted to medications that lower the blood glucose, but diabetes involves more than elevated blood glucose levels. People with diabetes often have high blood pressure and high cholesterol, and they suffer more sickness when exposed to influenza or pneumonia. It is important to consider this fact in the overall management of your disease.

If you have high blood pressure, lifestyle changes, including weight loss and physical activity, may be all you need to control the condition. However, if lifestyle changes alone don't work, numerous medications are available that control blood pressure. See my book *High Blood Pressure For Dummies* (Wiley) for a complete discussion of this subject. Controlling blood pressure is as important as controlling blood glucose in preventing diabetic complications.

Most people with diabetes also have elevated levels of LDL or "bad" cholesterol. Excellent drugs are available to manage this problem if lifestyle changes don't suffice. See *Controlling Cholesterol For Dummies* (Wiley) by Carol Ann Rinzler and Martin W. Graf for the answers to your questions on this topic. Cholesterol control is another cornerstone of excellent diabetic care.

People with diabetes, especially those whose glucose is poorly controlled, are prone to become sicker when they develop influenza or pneumonia. Excellent vaccinations for these illnesses are available. Flu vaccine is given annually, and pneumonia vaccine is given once if you are older than 65 and received a previous vaccination more than five years ago.

Finally, aspirin has been shown to reduce sickness and death due to coronary artery disease. Because coronary artery disease is such a prominent feature of diabetes, many doctors recommend that all patients with diabetes take a daily aspirin tablet. Diabetics may need more than the usual dose of a baby aspirin to reduce their risk of heart attacks; a full adult pill may be necessary.

Avoiding Drug Interactions

Studies have shown that some patients with diabetes are taking as many as four to five drugs, including their diabetes medications. These drugs often interact, and the cost of treating harmful drug interactions is more than $4 billion. Sometimes (believe it or not) even your doctor is not aware of the interactions of common drugs. You need to know the names of all the drugs you take and whether they affect one another.

 You should never take a drug, or a combination of drugs, as a convenient way of avoiding the basic diet and exercise that are the keys to diabetic control. (See Chapters 6 and 7 for more information on these crucial points.)

 Many common medications used for the treatment of high blood pressure also raise the blood glucose, sometimes bringing out a diabetic tendency that might otherwise not have been recognized:

✔ **Thiazide diuretics** often raise the glucose by causing a loss of potassium. Among these drugs are Diuril, hydroDiuril, Oretic, and Zaroxolyn.

✔ **Beta blockers** reduce the release of insulin and include such drugs as Inderal, Lopressor, and Tenormin.

✔ **Calcium channel blockers** also reduce insulin secretion and include Adalat, Calan, Cardizem, Isoptin, Norvasc, and Procardia.

✔ **Minoxidil** can raise blood glucose.

Drugs used for other purposes can also raise blood glucose:

✔ **Corticosteroids,** even in topical use, can raise blood glucose.

✔ **Cyclosporine,** used to prevent organ rejection, can raise the blood glucose by poisoning the insulin-producing beta cell.

✔ **Diphenylhydantoin,** known as Dilantin, is a drug for seizures and blocks insulin release.

✔ **Nicotinic acid and niacin,** used to lower cholesterol, can bring out a hyperglycemic tendency.

✔ **Oral contraceptives** were previously accused of causing hyperglycemia when the dose of estrogen was very high, but current preparations are not a problem.

✔ **Phenothiazines,** such as Compazine, Serentil, Stelazine, and Thorazine, can block insulin secretion and cause hyperglycemia.

✔ **Thyroid hormone,** in elevated levels, raises the blood glucose by reducing insulin from the pancreas.

Many common medications, either on their own or by doing something to make the oral drugs that lower blood glucose more potent, also lower the blood glucose. The most important of these include the following:

✔ **Salicylates and acetaminophen,** known as aspirin and Tylenol, can lower the blood glucose, especially when given in large doses.

✔ **Ethanol,** in any form of alcohol, can lower the blood glucose, particularly when taken without food.

✔ **Angiotensin converting enzyme inhibitors,** used for high blood pressure, such as Accupril, Captopril, Lotensin, Monopril, Prinivil, Vasotec, and Zestril, can lower the blood glucose, though the mechanism is unclear.

✔ **Alpha-blockers,** another group of antihypertensives that includes Prazosin, lower the glucose as well.

✔ **Fibric acid derivatives** like Clofibrate, used to treat disorders of fat, cause a lowering of blood glucose.

Finding Financial Assistance

Diabetes can be expensive, especially if you need several drugs to control your blood glucose. The pharmaceutical companies understand, and several offer programs to provide medication for a period of time:

✔ Bayer Corporation (acarbose), 800-998-9180

✔ Bristol-Myers Squibb (metformin), 800-437-0994

✔ Eli Lilly and Company (all insulin preparations), 800-545-6962

✔ Novo Nordisk (insulin preparations), 800-727-6500

✔ Pfizer (glipizide, glipizide extended release, chlorpropamide), 800-438-1985

✔ Sanofi-Aventis (glyburide, glimepiride, Lantus), 800-221-4025

All these programs require you to get a prescription from your doctor. The doctor usually fills out forms that state that the patient meets the financial requirements and needs the drug. Not all companies give away free drugs for life. If you cannot afford to buy a drug that you're taking, do not hesitate to call the company and ask whether it has a patient-assistance program.

Chapter 5

Using Insulin

*I*f you have type 1 diabetes, insulin is your savior. If you have type 2 diabetes, you may need insulin late in the course of your disease. Insulin is a great drug, but most people take it through a needle, and that is the rub (or the pain). Inventors have come up with many different ways to administer insulin, but using a syringe and a needle has been the standard for so long that most patients continue to do so. In this chapter, I tell you about those newer methods and about how and why you use insulin.

Checking Out Types of Insulin

In the human body, insulin is constantly responding to ups and downs in the blood glucose. No simple device is currently available to measure the blood glucose and give insulin as the pancreas does. (Check out Chapter 2 for more about the pancreas.) In order to avoid having to take many shots a day, forms of

insulin were invented to work at different times.
These forms of insulin include

✔ **Rapid-acting lispro insulin:** Lispro insulin
(called *Humalog insulin* by its manufacturer, Eli
Lilly) begins to lower the glucose within 5 minutes of administration, peaks at about one hour,
and is no longer active by about three hours.

Lispro is a great advance because it frees the
person with diabetes to take a shot just when he
or she eats. With the previous short-acting insulin (regular insulin), a person had to take a shot
and eat within 30 minutes or hypoglycemia
might occur. Because its activity begins and
ends so quickly, lispro does not cause hypoglycemia as often as the older preparations.

Novo Nordisk has come out with *insulin aspart*
(called NovoLog), which has characteristics
indistinguishable from lispro insulin.

✔ **Short-acting regular insulin:** Regular insulin
takes 30 minutes to start to lower the glucose,
peaks at 3 hours, and is gone by 6 to 8 hours.
Until Humalog and NovoLog came along,
patients used this preparation before meals to
keep their glucose low until the next meal.

✔ **Intermediate-acting NPH or Lente insulins:**
Both begin to lower the glucose within 2 hours
of administration and continue their activity for
10 to 12 hours. They can be active for up to 24
hours. This kind of insulin provides a smooth
level of control over half the day so that a low
level of active insulin is always in the body. This
attempts to parallel the situation that exists in
the human body.

✔ **Long-acting Ultralente insulin:** This insulin
begins to act within 6 hours and provides a low
level of insulin activity for up to 26 hours. It was
invented to provide a smooth, basal level of

control requiring only one shot a day. It can act differently in different people, looking more like intermediate insulin in some patients.

✔ **Long-acting insulin glargine and detemir:** Aventis sells an insulin called *insulin glargine* or Lantus. Studies have shown that insulin glargine has its onset in 1 to 2 hours after injection, and its activity lasts for 24 hours without a specific peak time of activity, which is exactly what is needed to control the blood glucose over an entire day.

Insulin glargine is released in a smooth fashion from the site of injection, and it doesn't matter what part of the body is injected. Because of its smooth and predictable activity, insulin glargine does not tend to cause low blood glucose at night, which often happens with NPH insulin. One disadvantage of insulin glargine is that it can't be mixed with other insulins in one syringe.

Insulin detemir or Levemir has similar properties to glargine but does not last quite as long. It is a product of Novo Nordisk.

If you don't have good diabetic control (defined as hemoglobin A1c of 7 percent or less) with NPH insulin, ask your doctor to consider using insulin glargine.

✔ **Premixed insulins:** Several mixtures are available: one with 70 percent NPH insulin and 30 percent regular; one with a 50–50 mix of NPH and regular; one with a 75–25 mix of NPH-like insulin and lispro insulin; and one with a 70–30 mix of NPH-like insulin and insulin aspart. These insulins are helpful for people who have trouble mixing insulins in one syringe, have poor eyesight, or are stable on a preparation that does not change.

Combining insulin and oral agents in type 2 diabetes

Sometimes the characteristics of the currently available oral agents (see Chapter 4) do not provide the tight control needed to avoid complications. This is particularly true after many years of type 2 diabetes. Then insulin may be required. Insulin may be added in a number of ways, but often a shot of glargine insulin at bedtime is all that you need to start the day under control and continue it with oral agents. For example, rosiglitazone may control the daytime glucoses very well after eating, but the first morning glucose may need the overnight shot of glargine insulin. By gradually increasing the dose of glargine, most patients with type 2 diabetes on oral agents can be controlled so that their hemoglobin A1c is 7 or below.

As type 2 diabetes progresses, the oral agents may be less effective, and insulin is taken more often. Two shots a day of intermediate and short-acting insulin may do the trick. Usually you take two-thirds of the dose in the morning and one-third before supper because you need short-acting insulin to control the supper carbohydrates.

You need to know a few things that are common to all insulins:

✔ Insulin may be kept at room temperature for four weeks or in the refrigerator until the expiration date printed on the label. After four weeks at room temperature, the insulin should be discarded.

✔ Insulin doesn't take too well to excessive heat, such as direct sunlight, or excessive cold. Protect your insulin against these conditions.

✔ You can safely give an insulin shot through clothing.

✔ If you take less than 50 units in a shot, there are ½ cc syringes that make it easy to measure up to 50 units. If you take less than 30 units, you can use ³⁄₁₀ cc syringes.

✔ Shorter needles may be more comfortable, especially for children, but the depth of the injection helps to determine how fast the insulin works.

✔ You can reuse disposable syringes a couple of times.

✔ Used syringes and needles must be disposed of in a puncture-proof container that is sealed shut before being placed in the trash.

Using a Syringe

Whatever type of insulin you use, chances are you'll be taking it by syringe and needle. Drawing insulin up is done in the same way no matter which type of insulin is involved. Starting at the needle end of the syringe, you'll find nine small lines above the needle, followed by a tenth longer line where the number 10 may be found. Each line is one unit of insulin. Above the 10-unit line, you'll find a succession of four small lines followed by a larger line representing 15, 20, 25, and so on.

If the insulin is lispro or regular, it should be clear, and you don't have to shake the bottle. The other kinds of insulin are cloudy, and you need to shake the bottle a few times to suspend the tiny particles in the liquid. When you're ready to take insulin, wipe the rubber stopper in the top of the bottle with alcohol.

Pull up the number of units of air that corresponds to the number of units of insulin you need to take. Turn the insulin bottle upside down and penetrate the rubber stopper with the needle of the syringe. Push all the air inside and pull out the insulin dose you need. Because air replaces the insulin, the pressure inside the bottle is unchanged, and no vacuum is created. Check to make sure that you have the right amount of the right insulin and no air bubbles in the syringe.

To give the injection, use alcohol to wipe off an area of skin on your arm, chest, stomach, or wherever you're injecting it. Insert the needle at a right angle to the skin and push it in. When the needle has penetrated the skin, push the plunger of the syringe down to zero to administer the insulin.

If you're taking two kinds of insulin at the same time (but not insulin glargine), you can mix them in one syringe, thus avoiding two shots. Here's how:

1. **Wipe both bottles with alcohol.**

2. **Draw up the total units of air corresponding to the total insulin you need.**

3. **Push the units of air into the longer-acting insulin bottle that correspond to the number of units of longer-acting insulin you need, and withdraw the needle.**

4. **Push the rest of the units of air into the shorter-acting insulin bottle, and withdraw the correct units of insulin.**

5. **Go back to the longer-acting bottle and withdraw the correct units of insulin from there.**

   By doing this, you do not contaminate the shorter-acting insulin with the additive in the longer-acting insulin.

Utilizing aids to insulin delivery

For those of you using the needle-and-syringe method, I want you to be aware of numerous aids that can make it easier for you to take insulin:

Spring-loaded syringe holders: You place your syringe in the holder, hold it against the skin, and press a button. The needle enters, and you've administered the insulin.

Syringe magnifiers: These help the visually impaired person administer insulin.

Syringe-filling devices: You can feel and hear a click as you take up insulin.

Subcutaneous infusion sets: A catheter is placed under the skin, and injections are made into the catheter instead of the skin to reduce punctures.

Needle guides: You can use these guides when you can't see the rubber part of the insulin bottle to insert the needle to take up the insulin.

Call your local American Diabetes Association branch or look in the back of the ADA's *Diabetes Forecast* magazine to find sources for these products.

Where you inject the insulin helps determine how fast it works. Insulin injected into the abdomen is most rapidly absorbed, followed by the arms and legs and then the buttocks. You may use these differing rates of uptake of the insulin to get faster action when your blood glucose is high. If the body part that gets the insulin is exercised, the insulin enters more quickly. If you use the same injection site repeatedly, the absorption rate slows down, so rotate the sites.

The timing of your insulin injections helps to determine the smoothness of your glucose control. The more regular you are in your injections, your eating, and your exercise, the smoother your glucose level.

Conducting Intensive Insulin Treatment

Intensive insulin treatment is essential in type 1 diabetes if you hope to prevent the complications of the disease. This means measuring your blood glucose at least before each meal and at bedtime, plus using both short-acting and longer-acting insulin to keep the blood glucose between 80 and 100 before meals and less than 140 after eating. How you do this is the subject of this section.

In a person who doesn't have type 1 diabetes, a small amount of circulating insulin is always present in the bloodstream and increases temporarily after the person eats to control the glucose in the meal. Intensive insulin treatment attempts to mirror the activity of the normal human pancreas as much as possible.

In intensive insulin treatment, you usually take a certain amount of longer-acting insulin at bedtime. I prefer insulin glargine because it produces a smooth basal level of glucose control over 24 hours. In addition, you take a dose of rapid-acting insulin before each meal. I prefer lispro because it is more convenient and less hypoglycemia occurs.

The dose of lispro is determined by the expected grams of carbohydrates in the meal you're about to eat, as well as by your blood glucose at that moment. Your doctor should provide you with a list of how much insulin to take for a given situation.

Using the carbohydrates in a meal to determine your insulin dose is called *carbohydrate counting*. The key to this system is to know the carbohydrates in your food. Here is where you make use of your friendly dietitian, who can go over your food preferences and show you how many carbohydrates are in them. The dietitian can also show you where to find carbohydrate counts for any other foods that you might eat.

You also need to know how many grams of carbohydrate are controlled by each unit of insulin you take. This is determined by checking your blood glucose an hour after eating a known amount of carbohydrate. For example, one person may need 1 unit to control 20 grams of carbohydrate, while another person needs 1 unit to control 15 grams of carbohydrate. If both of them eat a breakfast of 75 grams of carbohydrate, the first person might take 4 units of lispro, while the second person takes 5 units of lispro. Then additional units are added for the amount that the blood glucose needs to be lowered.

A typical schedule is to take 1 unit for every 50 mg/dl that the blood glucose is above 100 mg/dl. Insulin can also be subtracted if the blood glucose is too low. For every 50 mg/dl that the glucose is below 100, subtract 1 unit. By measuring your blood glucose frequently, you can find out how different carbohydrates affect your blood glucose. By using the carbohydrate sources that have a low glycemic index, you will need to use less insulin to control them. (See Chapter 6 for more on carbohydrates.)

As you attempt to help your body mirror normal insulin and glucose dynamics, you often have to deal with a greater frequency of hypoglycemia. The best way to handle hypoglycemia is by eating slightly smaller meals and using the unused calories as between-meal snacks. This technique smooths out the ups and downs.

At what point do you adjust your insulin glargine? If you find that several mornings in a row your fasting blood glucose is too high, you might add a unit or two to your bedtime glargine. If it's too low, you might reduce your insulin glargine by a unit or two or try eating a small bedtime snack. A high blood glucose level throughout the day is an indication to raise the glargine. Getting a lot of hypoglycemia at different times of day is a reason to lower the glargine.

These adjustments are best done in consultation with your doctor. If, however, you're unable to see your doctor, you can put your knowledge to use and make these adjustments on your own.

Investigating Other Methods for Delivering Insulin

Syringes have been used to deliver insulin since the beginning, but one of the newer methods for delivering insulin may be worth considering.

Delivering insulin with a pen

Several manufacturers have sought ways to make delivering insulin easier. The insulin pen is one useful tool. It doesn't eliminate the need for needles, but it does change the way you measure your insulin. Either the pen comes with an insulin cartridge already inserted, or the cartridge is placed inside the pen just like ink cartridges used to be put in pens.

You can dial the amount of insulin that you need to take. Each unit (sometimes two units) is accompanied by a clicking sound so the visually impaired can hear the number of units. The units also appear in a window on the pen. If you draw up too many units, one of the pens forces you to waste the insulin by pushing it out of the needle, while others allow you to reset the pen and start again. Depending on the pen, you can deliver from 30 to 70 units of insulin. You screw on a new needle as needed.

 The most commonly used pens are made by Eli Lilly and Novo Nordisk. Patients tell me that whether they use the Eli Lilly or the Novo Nordisk pen, the Novo Fine Pen Needles are less painful.

Should you shift from your syringe and needle to a pen? If you're comfortable with the syringe and needle and feel your technique is accurate, you probably have no reason to do so. If you're new to insulin, have some visual impairment, or feel that you're not getting an accurate measurement of the insulin, a pen may be the solution for you.

Delivering insulin with a jet injection device

Jet injection devices are for the person who just can't stick a needle into his or her skin. At around $1,000 or more, they're expensive, but they last a long time and replace the syringe and needle.

A large quantity of insulin is taken into the injection device, enough for multiple treatments. The amount of insulin to be delivered is measured, usually by rotating one part of the device while the number of units to be delivered appears in a window. The device is held against the skin. With the press of a button, a powerful jet of air forces the insulin through the skin into the subcutaneous tissue, usually with no pain perceived by the patient. The devices come in a lower power form for smaller children. These devices can deliver up to 50 units at one time.

Should you try an insulin jet injector? If you have no
trouble with the syringe and needle or find the pen to
be an easy substitute, you don't need a jet injector. If
you hate needles or need to give frequent shots to a
small child who is very resistant to them, a jet injector may solve your problems.

Delivering insulin with an external pump

For some people — and you may be one of them —
the external insulin pump is the answer to their
prayers. These devices are as close as you currently
can come to the gradual administration of rapid-
acting insulin that is normally taking place in the
body. They're expensive, costing more than $4,000,
but the insulin pump may be the answer for patients
who simply cannot achieve good glucose control with
syringes, pens, or jet injectors.

Pumps are the size of a pager. Inside is a motor. A
syringe filled with short-acting insulin is placed within
the pump, with the plunger against a screw that
slowly pushes it down to push insulin out of the
syringe. The end of the syringe is attached to a short
tube, which ends in a needle pushed into the skin of
the abdomen. Insulin is slowly pushed under the skin.

The rate at which insulin slowly enters the abdomen
is called the *basal rate*. It can be set, by way of computer chips, to vary as often as every half hour to an
hour. For example, from 8 a.m. to 9 a.m., the pump
may deliver 0.8 units, while from 9 a.m. to 10 a.m., the
pump may deliver 1.0 units, depending upon the
needs of the patient. This amount is determined, of
course, by measuring the blood glucose with a meter
(see Chapter 3).

When the patient is about to eat a meal, he or she can push a button to deliver extra insulin, called a *bolus* of insulin. (The amount is determined by carbohydrate counting, which I explain earlier in this chapter.) You can get extra insulin if the blood glucose is too high at any time.

Pump usage is definitely not treatment to be done on your own at the beginning. You need a diabetologist to help with dosages, a dietitian to help you calculate amounts of boluses based upon carbohydrate intake, and someone from the manufacturer to teach you how to set the pump and to be available to fix any malfunctions.

Is an insulin pump for you? If you're willing to invest the time and effort at first, if your schedule is very uncertain particularly with respect to meals, and if your glucose control has not been good with other means, you should look into this option.

My patients who use the pump have generally had positive experiences. Now that they have it, none of them are willing to give up the pump. Occasionally, they disconnect the pump to allow their skin to heal. They have generally shown improved glucose control and a better hemoglobin A1c.

Chapter 6

Looking Into a Diabetes Diet Plan

. . . .

In This Chapter

▶ Knowing how many kilocalories to consume

▶ Monitoring carbohydrates, glycemic index, and fiber

▶ Picking the best proteins and fats

▶ Getting enough vitamins, minerals, and water

▶ Using sweeteners other than sugar

▶ Discovering dietary needs of type 1 and type 2 diabetes

▶ Looking at weight loss considerations

. . . .

*A*re you watching your weight go higher and higher? Do you think that *low calorie* refers to the food on the bottom shelf of the supermarket?

For the diabetic population, most of whom are overweight, appropriate nutrition and weight loss are not an option but a necessity. In this chapter, you find out all you need to know to make your diet work for you, not only to improve your diabetes and control your blood glucose, but to generally feel that you have an improved quality of life.

Considering Total Calories First

No matter how you slice it, your weight is determined by the number of calories you take in, minus the number of calories you use up by exercise or loss of calories in the urine or bowel movements. If you have an excess of calories coming in and have insulin with which to store them, you gain weight. If you have fewer calories in than out, you lose weight. If you are overweight, you benefit from even a small weight loss:

- ✔ Weight loss markedly reduces the risk of developing type 2 diabetes.

- ✔ Weight loss prevents the progression of prediabetes (see Chapter 1) into type 2 diabetes.

- ✔ Weight loss can reverse the failure to respond to drugs for diabetes that develops after responding at first.

- ✔ Weight loss reduces the risk of death from diabetes.

- ✔ Weight loss increases life expectancy in patients with type 2 diabetes.

- ✔ Weight loss has beneficial effects on high blood pressure and abnormal fats.

A study of portion sizes between 1977 and 1998, which was published in the *Journal of the American Medical Association* in January 2003, showed that portion sizes have increased dramatically, especially in fast food restaurants and at home. One simple and effective way to cut your calories is to eat half to two-thirds of what you're served and save the rest for another time.

To have an approximate idea of how many *kcalories* (kilocalories) you need each day (not *calories,* which are much smaller), you need to figure your desirable weight. A 5-foot 6-inch male with a moderate frame should weigh around 142 pounds. To find the number of kcalories needed:

1. **Multiply your weight times 10.** In our example, this gives a value of about 1,400 kcalories.

2. **Add kcalories for your level of exercise:**

   A sedentary male adds 10 percent of the basal kcalories.

   A moderately active male adds 20 percent.

   A very active male adds 40 percent or more, depending on the length and the degree of exercise.

If the male in our example is moderately active, he needs 1,400 kcalories plus 1,400 times 20 percent (or about 300) more for a total of 1,700 kcalories.

 These formulas are true for women as well, but women usually require fewer kcalories to maintain the same weight as men. Be aware that this is an approximation that differs not only for different people but even for the same person on different days.

When you determine the total kcalories you need, the question becomes how to divide the calories among various foods. Basically, three types of foods contain calories: Carbohydrates, proteins, and fats. Within these foods, you have many variables, which I explain in the following sections.

Carbohydrates

There's no more controversial area in nutrition for the diabetic person than carbohydrates. In this section, I give you my suggestions for carbohydrate in your diet based on my reading of the medical literature and my clinical experience. You are free to disagree with me and use whatever level of carbohydrate you like as long as it helps to promote a lower blood glucose without increasing your blood fats or weight.

Carbohydrates are the sources of energy that start with *glucose,* the sugar in your bloodstream that's one sugar molecule, and include substances containing many sugar molecules called *complex carbohydrates, starches, cellulose,* and *gums.* Some of the common sources of carbohydrate are bread, potatoes, grains, cereals, and rice.

Physicians know a lot of information about carbohydrate in the body:

- ✔ Carbohydrate is the primary source of energy for muscles.
- ✔ Glucose is the carbohydrate that causes the pancreas to release insulin.
- ✔ Carbohydrate causes the triglyceride (fat) level to rise in the blood.
- ✔ When insulin isn't present or is ineffective, more carbohydrate raises the blood glucose higher.
- ✔ If simple sugars are in the diet in increased amounts, they aren't harmful as long as the total calorie count is satisfactory.

Because carbohydrate is the food that raises the blood glucose, which is responsible for the complications of diabetes, it seems right to recommend a diet that's lower in carbohydrate than previously suggested.

 My experience has been that a diet of 40 percent carbohydrate makes controlling blood glucose much easier. It also leads to weight loss because you don't tend to substitute protein or fat for the reduced amount of carbohydrate in the diet.

My patients on lower carbohydrate diets are able to reduce the amounts of drugs they take, such as insulin, which can cause weight gain and complicate controlling their diabetes. They also have a better fat profile.

All carbohydrates are not alike in the degree to which they raise the blood glucose. This fact was recognized some years ago, and a measurement called the glycemic index was created to quantify it.

The *glycemic index* (GI) uses white bread as the indicator food and assigns it a value of 100. Another carbohydrate of equal calories is compared to white bread in its ability to raise the blood glucose and is assigned a value in comparison to white bread. A food that raises glucose half as much as white bread has a GI of 50, while a food that raises glucose 1½ times as much has a GI of 150.

The point is to select carbohydrates with low GI levels to try to keep the glucose response as low as possible. A glycemic index of 70 or more is high; 56 to 69 is medium; and 55 or less is low.

I believe that switching to low GI carbohydrates can be very beneficial for controlling the glucose. You can easily make some simple substitutions in your diet, as shown in Table 6-1.

Table 6-1	Low-GI Diet Substitutions
High-GI Food	*Low-GI Food*
Whole meal or white bread	Whole grain bread
Processed breakfast cereal	Unrefined cereals like oats or processed low GI cereals

(continued)

Table 6-1 *(continued)*

High-GI Food	Low-GI Food
Plain cookies and crackers	Cookies made with dried fruits or whole grains like oats
Cakes and muffins	Cakes and muffins made with fruit, oats, and whole grains
Tropical fruits like bananas	Temperate climate fruits like apples and plums
Potatoes	Pasta or legumes
Rice	Basmati or other low GI rice

Fiber is the part of the carbohydrate that isn't digestible and, therefore, adds no calories. Fiber is found in most fruits, grains, and vegetables. Fiber comes in two forms:

- ✔ **Soluble fiber:** This form of fiber can dissolve in water and has a lowering effect on blood glucose and fat levels, particularly cholesterol.

- ✔ **Insoluble fiber:** This form of fiber cannot dissolve in water and remains in the intestine. It absorbs water and stimulates movement in the intestine. Insoluble fiber also helps prevent constipation and possibly colon cancer. This is the fiber called *bulk* or *roughage*.

Before the current trend to refine foods, people ate many sources of carbohydrate that were high in fiber. These were all in plant foods, such as fruits, vegetables, and grains. Animal foods contain no fiber.

The way to eat the right amount of carbohydrate without increasing your blood glucose or triglycerides is to make it a low-glycemic, high-fiber carbohydrate.

Proteins

Your choice of protein is very important because some is very high in fat while some is relatively fat-free. The following lists can give you an idea of the fat content of various sources of protein.

One ounce of **very lean** meat, fish, or substitutes has 7 grams of protein and 1 gram of fat. Examples include

- Skinless white meat chicken or turkey
- Flounder, halibut, or tuna canned in water
- Lobster, shrimp, or clams
- Fat-free cheese

An ounce of **lean** meat, fish, or substitutes has 7 grams of protein and 3 grams of fat. Examples include

- Lean beef, lean pork, lamb, or veal
- Dark meat chicken without skin or white meat chicken with skin
- Sardines, salmon, or tuna canned in oil
- Other meats or cheeses with 3 grams of fat per ounce

An ounce of **medium-fat** meat, fish, or substitutes has 7 grams of protein plus 5 grams of fat. Examples include

- Most beef products
- Regular fat pork, lamb, or veal
- Dark meat chicken with skin or fried chicken
- Fried fish
- Cheeses with 5 grams of fat per ounce, such as feta and mozzarella

High-fat meat, fish, or substitutes contain 8 grams of fat and 7 grams of protein per ounce. Examples include

- ✔ Pork spareribs or pork sausage
- ✔ Bacon
- ✔ Regular cheeses like cheddar and Monterey Jack
- ✔ Processed sandwich meats

A lot of controversy exists with regard to how much protein should be in the diet. Many authorities call for less than 30 percent, usually preferring a diet that has 20 percent of calories as protein. One reason has to do with the large fat content of some protein sources. However, if you select protein with less fat, you can solve that problem.

My recommendation is that 30 percent of your kcalories come from protein.

Fats

The amount of fat you need is a lot less controversial than the carbohydrate and protein in your diet. Everyone agrees that you should eat no more than 30 percent of your diet as fats. (Currently, the U.S. population eats 36 percent of its diet as fats.)

Keep in mind that some fats are more dangerous in their tendency to promote coronary artery disease than others. These fats should make up less of the dietary fat than the safer fats.

Cholesterol is the fat everyone knows. It has been shown to be the culprit in the development of coronary artery disease, as well as peripheral vascular disease and cerebrovascular disease.

Protein chemistry

Just as most carbohydrate contains no protein, most protein contains no carbohydrate. Therefore, protein does not raise blood glucose levels significantly under normal circumstances.

When the protein enters the small intestine, it is broken down into the smaller molecules of amino acids of which it is made. The amino acids are absorbed into the bloodstream and head for the liver, where some are converted into glucose. This means dietary protein can raise glucose, but this process takes place slowly and isn't a major contributor to the blood glucose. Some of the amino acids are used to build new protein.

The recommendation is that no more than 300 milligrams a day of fat come from cholesterol. One egg can take care of that prescription. Most other foods that you eat regularly don't contain a lot of cholesterol, but whole milk and hard cheeses like cheddar contain saturated fat, which raises the cholesterol in the body.

The other kind of fat is triglyceride, which comes in several forms:

✔ **Saturated fat** is the kind of fat that usually comes from animal sources. The streaks of fat in a steak are saturated fat. Butter is made up of saturated fat. Bacon, cream, and cream cheese are other examples. Vegetable sources of saturated fat include coconut, palm, and palm kernel oils. Eating a lot of saturated fat increases your blood cholesterol level.

✔ **Trans fatty acid** is produced when polyunsatu-rated fat (which I describe in the next bullet) is heated and hydrogen is bubbled through it. Fully hydrogenated, it becomes solid fat; par-tially hydrogenated, it has a consistency like butter and can be used in its place. Food manu-facturers have used trans fatty acids to replace butter because trans fatty acids are cheaper.

Trans fatty acids may contribute more to the development of heart disease than saturated fats. Keep them out of your diet! The govern-ment now requires food labels to list trans fats, so read those labels.

✔ **Unsaturated fat** comes from vegetable sources like olive oil, canola oil, and margarine. Monounsaturated fat (as in avocado and olive oil) does not raise cholesterol. Polyunsaturated fat (like corn oil or margarine) doesn't raise cho-lesterol but causes a reduction in the good or HDL cholesterol.

Keeping in mind that 30 percent of your total daily calories should come from fat, less than a third of that amount should come from saturated fats. You should also keep your dietary cholesterol under 300 milligrams per day.

Getting Enough Vitamins, Minerals, and Water

Your diet must contain sufficient vitamins and miner-als, but the amount you need may be less than you think. If you eat a balanced diet that comes from the various food groups, you generally get enough vita-mins for your daily needs.

Counting alcohol as part of your diet

Because alcohol has calories, if you drink some, you must account for it in your diet. The *proof* of the alcohol is the percentage of alcohol in an ounce of the drink multiplied by 2. Wine that is 12.5 percent alcohol is 25 proof. Beer is 12 proof most of the time. Liquor is often 80 proof. To determine the calories, use the following formula:

Calories = 0.8 x proof of the drink x number of ounces

So, for example, for a 12-ounce can of beer, you use the formula 0.8 x 12 x 12 for a total of 115 kilocalories.

For a couple of 6-ounce glasses of wine, you use the formula 0.8 x 25 x 12 to come up with 240 kilocalories.

In addition to the calories, alcohol plays other roles in diabetes. If alcohol is taken without food, it can cause low blood glucose by increasing the activity of insulin without food to compensate for it. Some alcoholics, even without diabetes, go to bed with several drinks in their systems and are unconscious the next morning because of very low blood glucose. They can have brain damage unless their bodies are able to manufacture enough glucose to wake them up.

If you're having a couple glasses of wine or other alcohol, make sure that you eat some food with it.

In certain situations, such as if you are pregnant, you need to be sure that you are getting enough every day, so you take a vitamin supplement. Some evidence also suggests that extra vitamin C protects against colds.

As far as the other vitamins go, the proof just does not exist that large amounts of the vitamins are beneficial, and in some cases, they may be harmful. I do not recommend that you take megadoses of these vitamins.

Minerals are also key ingredients of a healthy diet. Most are needed in tiny amounts, which are easily consumed from a balanced diet.

Water is the last important nutrient I discuss in this section, but it is by no means the least important. Your body is made up of 60 percent or more water. All the nutrients in the body are dissolved in water. You can live without food for some time, but you will not last long without water.

 Water can help to give a feeling of fullness that reduces appetite. In general, people don't drink enough water. You need to drink a minimum of 10 cups, or 2½ quarts, of water a day.

Using Sugar Substitutes

Fear of the "danger" of sugar in the diet has led to a vast effort to produce a compound that can add the pleasurable sweetness without the liabilities of sugar. Interestingly enough, despite the availability of a number of excellent sweeteners, some containing no calories at all, the incidence of diabetes continues to rise. Still, if you can reduce your caloric intake or your glucose response by using a sweetener, doing so has advantages. Sweeteners are divided into those that contain calories and those that do not.

Among the calorie-containing sweeteners are

✔ **Fructose, found in fruits and berries:** Fructose is actually sweeter than table sugar *(sucrose)*. However, it's absorbed more slowly from the intestine than glucose, so it raises the blood glucose more slowly. It's taken up by the liver and converted to glucose or triglycerides.

✔ **Xylitol, found in strawberries and raspberries:** Xylitol is about like fructose in terms of sweetness. It's taken up slowly from the intestine so that it causes little change in blood glucose. Xylitol doesn't cause cavities of the teeth as often as the other sweeteners containing calories, so it's used in chewing gum.

✔ **Sorbitol and mannitol, sugar alcohols occurring in plants:** Sorbitol and mannitol are half as sweet as table sugar and have little effect on blood glucose. They change to fructose in the body. When taken as a food, sorbitol doesn't accumulate and damage tissues.

The non-nutritive or artificial sweeteners are often much more sweet than table sugar — sometimes thousands of times sweeter. Therefore, much less of them is required to accomplish the same level of sweetness as sugar. The current artificial sweeteners include saccharin, aspartame, acesulfame, and sucralose.

For people with diabetes, recommendations regarding using sugar have been changed so that some sugar is permitted. The point is to count the calories eaten as sugar and subtract that from your permissible intake. If you do this, you'll have little use for either nutritive or the non-nutritive sweeteners.

Eating Well for Type 1 Diabetes

A person with type 1 diabetes takes insulin (see Chapter 5) to control the blood glucose. At this time, doctors and their patients cannot match the human pancreas in the way that it releases insulin just when the food is entering the bloodstream so that the glucose remains between 80 and 120 mg/dl. Therefore, the diabetic patient needs to make sure that his or her food enters as close to the expected activity of the insulin as possible.

Most people with type 1 diabetes take two different types of insulin: one that acts soon after the injection and has a brief period of activity, and a second that acts more slowly and lasts longer. The rapid-acting insulin is meant to cover the food eaten at meals, while the slower acting insulin covers the rest of the time, particularly overnight when a lot of circumstances tend to raise the blood glucose.

Fortunately, you can take a new type of insulin when you start to eat or even in the middle or at the end of a meal. This insulin overcomes the problem that always previously existed — that the shot had to be taken 30 minutes before eating to give it time to be active. A person with diabetes who had a meal delayed for any reason could easily become hypoglycemic using the old preparation.

The person with type 1 diabetes needs to be very careful when drinking alcohol. Alcohol increases the activity of insulin and can bring the blood glucose way down if food isn't taken with it. (See the sidebar on "Counting alcohol as part of your diet," earlier in this chapter.)

Because the person with type 1 diabetes always has some injected insulin circulating whether food is available or not, this patient shouldn't miss a meal. A midmorning snack and a midafternoon snack, and even a bedtime snack, if necessary, are particularly good ideas.

The person with type 1 diabetes needs to be willing to test the blood glucose frequently. That way, he or she can identify problems in advance. If, for example, your blood glucose is low before exercise, you can take some nutrition to avoid hypoglycemia.

Eating Well for Type 2 Diabetes

Because most people with type 2 diabetes are over-weight, weight control and reduction should be the major consideration. (See the next section for specific techniques to lose weight.)

The benefits of weight loss are rapidly seen, even when relatively little has been lost. The blood glucose falls rapidly. The blood pressure declines. The cholesterol falls. The triglycerides drop, and the good cholesterol (HDL) rises. Even a modest reduction of 10 percent of body weight has a significant positive effect on coronary artery disease.

 The person with type 2 diabetes has to be very aware of the fats in his or her diet. The metabolic syndrome is commonly found in this type of diabetes. You must pay attention to foods that increase triglycerides, which lead to the production of small, dense LDL particles that are connected to coronary artery disease.

Because hypertension is so prevalent in both types of diabetes and it makes diabetic complications occur earlier, reduction of salt intake is another important consideration.

Reducing Your Weight

Weight reduction is difficult for many reasons. In my experience, most patients do very well initially but tend to return to old habits. There's evidence that this tendency to regain weight is built into the human brain. When fat tissue is decreased or even increased, a central control system in the brain acts to restore the fat to the previous level. If liposuction is done, for example, the remaining cells swell up to hold more fat.

Mathematics of weight loss

A pound of fat contains 3,500 kcalories. In order to lose a pound of fat, therefore, you must eat 3,500 kcalories less than you need. You can do this by a daily reduction of 500 kcalories or by doing 200 kcalories extra of exercise daily and reducing the diet by only 300 kcalories per day. Using the first method, a man eating 1,700 kcalories per day needs to decrease his diet to 1,200.

Still, losing weight and keeping it off is possible. At one time, it was calculated that only 1 out of 20 people who lost weight would keep it off. Now the figure is closer to 1 out of 5.

In the next chapter, I cover the value of exercise in a weight loss program. At this point, you need to realize that successful maintenance of weight loss requires a willingness to make exercise a part of your daily life. If, for some reason, you cannot move your legs to exercise, you can get a satisfactory workout using your upper body alone. A recent study showed that 92 percent of people who maintain weight loss exercise regularly, while only 34 percent of those who regain their weight continue to exercise.

Types of diets

The numerous methods that are available for weight loss certainly suggest that no one method is especially better than all the rest. Some are fairly drastic in the degree to which they cut calories, and weight loss is fairly rapid. But these methods are particularly prone to result in restoration of the original weight.

Several diets are associated with large organizations and may require that you purchase only their foods. The support given by these organizations seems to be extremely helpful in weight-loss maintenance. In addition, the slower loss of weight and the connection to more normal eating seems to result in a greater tendency to stay with the program and keep the weight off. The leading contenders for this type of diet are Jenny Craig and Weight Watchers.

Do any of these diets have an advantage over the others? Researchers at the Pennsylvania School of Medicine put four groups of overweight people on four different popular diets — Atkins, Ornish, Weight Watchers, and the Zone — for a year. The result was that those people who stuck with the diet about 5 percent of their body weight, with no diet performing better than any other. Does that depress you? It shouldn't, because even that modest weight loss was associated with a 7 to 15 percent reduction of the risk of heart disease.

Behavior modification

Years of working with obese patients have shown me that weight loss requires more than a commitment to a sound diet and routine exercise; it requires changes in behavior with respect to food.

To lose weight and keep it off, you must change your eating behavior to make your diet easier to follow. Some of the best techniques include the following:

✔ Eat according to a schedule to avoid unplanned eating.

✔ Find a single place to eat all food.

✔ Slow down your eating to make the meal last.

✔ Put high-calorie foods away. Remove serving dishes and bread from the table.

✔ Don't dispense food to others to avoid exposure for yourself.

✔ Do not clean your plate.

✔ Set realistic goals for weight loss.

✔ When eating out, be careful of salad dressing, alcohol, and bread.

✔ Get a 10-pound weight and carry it around for a while to appreciate the importance of losing even that little.

✔ At the market, buy from a list, carry only enough money for the food on that list, and avoid aisles containing loose foods, other than fruits and vegetables, like loose candy.

Incorporate one technique into your life until you feel you have mastered it and have added it to your eating style. Then go on and take up another technique.

As you go about this difficult task of losing weight and keeping it off, remember to seek the help of those around you. A loving partner provides great help through the roughest days.

In an effort to lose weight, some people with diabetes skip their insulin shots. If you do so, your body will turn to fat for fuel because glucose can't be used, and you will lose weight. However, the result is that you also lose muscle mass, and your blood glucose rises very high. This is a dangerous situation and not a healthy approach to weight loss.

Chapter 7

Keeping It Moving: An Exercise Plan

. . . .

In This Chapter

▶ Understanding the importance of exercise

▶ Tailoring exercise for type 1 and type 2 patients

▶ Determining how long and how hard to exercise

▶ Choosing your activity

. . . .

M ore than 60 years ago, the great leaders in diabetes care declared that diabetes management has three major aspects:

✔ Proper diet

✔ Appropriate medication

✔ Sufficient exercise

Since then, millions of dollars and man (and woman) hours have been spent to define the proper diet and the right medication, but exercise has rarely received its proper place in the triad of care. I'm writing this chapter to correct that omission.

Getting Off the Couch: Why Exercise Is Essential

When the diabetes experts wrote recommendations for proper care, the isolation and administration of insulin had just recently begun, and they were focusing specifically on how to control type 1 diabetes. Since that time, many studies have shown that exercise doesn't normalize the blood glucose or reduce the hemoglobin A1c (see Chapter 3) in type 1 diabetes. Many other studies have shown that exercise does normalize blood glucose and reduce hemoglobin A1c in type 2 diabetes.

But while exercise cannot replace medication for the type 1 diabetic, its benefits are crucial for patients with both types of diabetes.

Preventing macrovascular disease

The major benefit of exercise for both types of diabetes is to prevent *macrovascular disease* (heart attack, stroke, or diminished blood flow to the legs). Macrovascular disease affects everyone, whether they have diabetes or not, but is particularly severe in people with diabetes. Exercise prevents macrovascular disease in numerous ways:

- ✔ Exercise helps with weight loss, which is especially important in type 2 diabetes.

- ✔ Exercise lowers bad cholesterol and triglycerides, and it raises good cholesterol.

- ✔ Exercise lowers blood pressure.

- ✔ Exercise lowers stress levels.

- ✔ Exercise reduces the need for insulin or drugs.

Understanding your body mechanics during exercise

The feeling of fatigue that occurs with exercise is probably due to the loss of stored muscle glucose. One way to preserve glucose stores is to provide calories from an external source. Any marathoner knows that additional calories can delay the feeling of exhaustion. The timing is important. If the glucose is given an hour before exercise, it will be metabolized during the exercise and increase endurance. However, if it's given 30 minutes before exercise, it may decrease stamina by stimulating insulin, which blocks liver production of glucose.

 Fructose can replenish you when you're doing prolonged exercise. This sweetener can replace glucose because it is sweeter but is absorbed more slowly and does not provoke the insulin secretion that glucose provokes. Fructose is rapidly converted into glucose inside the body.

Reaping the benefits

As your body becomes trained with regular exercise, the benefits for your diabetes are very significant. Your body starts to turn to fat for energy earlier in the course of your exercise. At the same time, the hormones that tend to raise the blood glucose during exercise are not produced at the same high rate because they aren't needed. Because you don't require as much insulin, your insulin doses can be reduced, and it's much easier to avoid hypoglycemia during exercise.

Exercising When You Have Diabetes

If you have diabetes and haven't exercised previously, you should check with a doctor prior to beginning a new exercise program, especially if you're over the age of 35 or if you've had diabetes for ten years or longer. You should also check with a doctor if you have any of the following risk factors:

- The presence of any diabetic complications like retinopathy, nephropathy, or neuropathy
- Obesity
- A physical limitation
- A history of coronary artery disease or elevated blood pressure
- Use of medications

When you begin to exercise, whether you have type 1 or type 2 diabetes, you can take many steps to make your experience safe and healthful. Some important steps to take include the following:

- Wear an ID bracelet.
- Test your blood glucose very often.
- Choose proper socks and shoes.
- Drink plenty of water.
- Carry treatment for hypoglycemia.
- Exercise with a friend.

Working out with type 1 diabetes

The person with type 1 diabetes depends on insulin injections to manage the blood glucose. He or she does not have the luxury of a "thermostat" that automatically shuts off during exercise and turns back on when exercise is finished. After an insulin shot is taken, it's active until it is used up.

 The person with type 1 diabetes has to avoid overdosing on insulin before exercise, which can lead to hypoglycemia, or underdosing, which can lead to hyperglycemia. If the body doesn't have enough insulin, it turns to fat for energy. Glucose rises because it isn't being metabolized but its production is continuing. If exercise is particularly vigorous in a situation of not enough insulin, the blood glucose can rise extremely high.

Reducing your insulin dosage prior to exercise helps prevent hypoglycemia. One study showed that an 80 percent reduction of the dose allowed the person with diabetes to exercise for 3 hours, while a 50 percent reduction forced the person with diabetes to stop after 90 minutes due to hypoglycemia. Each person with diabetes varies, and you must determine for yourself how much to reduce insulin by measuring the blood glucose before, during, and after exercise.

 Another way to prevent hypoglycemia, of course, is to eat some carbohydrate. You need to have some carbohydrate (which quickly raises blood glucose) available during exercise.

In addition, the site of the insulin injection is important because this determines how fast the insulin becomes active. If you are running and inject insulin into your leg, it will be taken up more quickly than an injection into the arm.

You can exercise whenever you will do it faithfully. If you like to sleep late and you schedule your exercise at 5:30 a.m., you probably won't consistently do it. Your best time to exercise is probably about 60 to 90 minutes after eating because this is when the glucose is peaking, providing the calories you need; if you exercise at this time you avoid the usual posteating high in your blood glucose, and you burn up those food calories.

Working out with type 2 diabetes

Other than the insulin discussion, many of the suggestions for the type 1 patient in the previous section apply to type 2 patients as well.

With sufficient exercise and diet, some people with type 2 diabetes can revert to a nondiabetic state. This does not mean that they no longer have diabetes but that they will not develop the long-term complications that can make them so miserable later in life.

Determining How Much Exercise to Do

Unless you have a physical abnormality, there is no limitation on what you can do. You need to select an activity that you enjoy and will continue to perform.

An hour (not an apple) a day keeps the doctor away! Moderate aerobic exercise done for an hour every day provides enormous physical, mental, and emotional benefits.

Exerting enough effort

In the recent past, exercise physiologists said that you needed to make sure that you monitored your exercise intensity by periodically checking your heart rate. Your exercise heart rate was supposed to be based on your age. The usual formula to figure this out is to take the number 220, subtract your age, and multiply that number by 60 to 75 percent to get the recommended exercise heart rate for aerobic exercise.

Now studies have shown that people can sustain aerobic exercise at higher heart rates. Perhaps the best way to know whether you're meeting your exercise goals is to use the "Perceived Exertion Scale" described in the sidebar "Checking the value of your exercise."

The younger you are, the faster your exercise heart rate may be. Like everything in this book, your exercise heart rate is an individual number. If you are a world-class athlete training for your ninth marathon, your exercise heart rate may be higher. If you have some heart disease, your exercise heart rate may be significantly lower.

Checking the value of your exercise

Measuring your pulse during exercise (or even at rest) may be hard for you. Instead, you can use the Perceived Exertion Scale. Exercise is given a descriptive value from *very, very light* to *very, very hard* with *very light, fairly light, somewhat hard,* and *very hard* in between. You want to exercise to a level of *somewhat hard,* and you will be at your target heart rate in most cases. As you get into shape, the amount of exertion that corresponds to *somewhat hard* will increase.

Do not continue exercising if you have tightness in your chest, chest pain, severe shortness of breath, or dizziness.

You need to warm up and cool down for about five minutes before and after you exercise. Stretching is one possibility for both warm-up and cool-down. If you do stretch, don't stretch to the point that it hurts. This is where muscle tears occur. See the excellent book *Fitness For Dummies,* 2nd Edition (Wiley), by Suzanne Schlosberg and Liz Neporent, M.A., for more about stretching.

Making moderate exercise your goal

Moderate exercise has a moving definition. If you're out of shape, moderate exercise for you may be slow walking. If you're in good shape, moderate exercise may be jogging or cross-country skiing. Moderate exercise is simply something you can do and not get out of breath. For ideas on the types of exercise you can do, see the following section.

How long can you stop exercise before you start to decondition? It takes only about two to three weeks to lose some of the fitness your exercise has provided. Then it takes up to six weeks to get back to your current level, assuming that your holiday from exercise does not go on too long.

Choosing an activity

Table 7-1 lists a variety of activities, including some that don't exactly fit into the category of *exercise* but offer some interesting comparisons. Next to each activity, I include the amount of kcalories that you burn in 20 minutes.

Table 7-1	Calories Burned in 20 Minutes	
Activity	*Kcalories Burned (125 pounds)*	*Kcalories Burned (175 pounds)*
Standing	24	32
Walking, 4 mph	104	144
Running, 7 mph	236	328
Gardening	60	84
Typing	38	54
Carpentry	64	88
House painting	58	80
Baseball	78	108
Dancing	70	96
Football	138	192
Golfing	66	96
Swimming	80	112
Skiing, downhill	160	224
Skiing, cross-country	196	276
Tennis	112	160

Your choice of an activity must take into account your physical condition:

✔ If you have diabetic neuropathy and cannot feel your feet, you do not want to do pounding exercises that may damage them without your awareness. You can swim, bike, row, or do arm-chair exercises where you move your upper body vigorously.

✔ If you have diabetic retinopathy, you won't want to do exercises that raise your blood pressure (like weight lifting), cause jerky motions in your eyes (like bouncing on a trampoline), or change the pressure in your eyes significantly (like scuba diving or high mountain climbing). You also shouldn't do exercises that place your eyes below the level of your heart, like toe touches.

✔ Patients with nephropathy should avoid exercises that raise the blood pressure for prolonged periods. These exercises are extremely intense activities that you do for a long time, like marathon running.

Some people have pain in the legs after they walk a certain distance. This may be due to diminished blood supply to the legs so that the needs of the muscles in the legs cannot be met. Although you need to discuss this problem with your doctor, you do not need to give up walking.

Instead, determine the distance you can walk up to the point of pain. Then walk about three-quarters of that distance and stop to give the circulation a chance to catch up. After you have rested, you will find that you can go about the same distance again without pain. By stringing several of these walks together, you can get a good, pain-free workout. You may even find that you are able to increase the distance after a while because this kind of training tends to create new blood vessels.

Is there a medical condition that should absolutely prevent you from doing exercise? Short of chest pain at rest, which must be addressed by your doctor, the answer is no.

If you can't figure out an exercise that you can do, get together with an exercise therapist. You'll be amazed at how many muscles you can move that you never knew you had.

When you need support

The Diabetes Exercise and Sports Association is an organization that you can turn to for help, instruction, and friendship as you add exercise to your good diabetes care. You can reach this organization by writing P.O. Box 1935, Litchfield Park, AZ 85340, or by calling 800-898-4322. They know all about diabetes and sports and are eager to share the information with you. See the Web site at `www.diabetes-exercise.org`.

Walking 10K a Day

The idea of walking 10,000 steps a day may seem like a huge, unattainable goal to you, but you may be surprised. This is certainly a goal worth striving toward because, as I discuss previously in this chapter, walking is one of the most beneficial exercises you can do.

The first step toward reaching this goal is to buy a *pedometer,* a device that you wear on your waist that counts each step you take.

Begin by doing your usual amount of exercise each day. Remember to record the steps at the end of the day and reset the button on the pedometer to zero. After seven days, add up the steps and divide by 7 to get your daily count. You will probably find that you are doing between 3,000 and 5,000 steps a day.

Next, you want to build up your daily number. Here are some tips to help:

✔ Get a good pair of walking shoes or sneakers and replace them when they begin to wear out.

✔ Leave your car parked. If you can make a trip in an hour or less by foot, save your gas money and add to your daily step count.

✔ Try to add a few hundred steps each week.

✔ Find an exercise buddy to walk with you. It's much more fun.

✔ Keep a record of the number of steps involved in various walks you take, so you can easily get the steps you're missing on any given day.

✔ Use stairs instead of the elevator, whether you're going up or down.

✔ Take a walk at lunchtime daily.

✔ Stop if you feel pain, and check with your doctor before continuing.

If you don't have a pedometer, or if you want to count other types of exercise toward your walking goal, use the following conversions:

✔ 1 mile = 2,100 average steps

✔ 1 block = 100 average steps

✔ 10 minutes walking = 1,200 steps on average

✔ Biking or swimming = 150 steps per minute

✔ Weight lifting = 100 steps per minute

✔ Rollerskating = 200 steps per minute

A study in the *Archives of Internal Medicine* in June 2003 provides the best evidence for the benefits of walking. Diabetics who walked at least two hours a week had a 40 percent lower death rate than inactive diabetics. What are you waiting for? Take the first steps!

Chapter 8

Ten Ways to Manage Diabetes

*I*f you read everything that came before this, congratulations. But I didn't expect that you would, and that's why I wrote this chapter. Follow the leader's (my) advice in this chapter, and you can be in great diabetic shape.

Major Monitoring

You have your glucose meter. Now what do you do with it? Most people don't like to stick themselves and are reluctant to do so at first. But you can monitor your glucose in so many ways, almost without pain, that you have no excuse for not doing so. How often you test is between you and your doctor, but the more you do it, the easier it is to control your diabetes. Monitoring gives you more insight into your particular body response to food, exercise, and medications. (See Chapter 3 for more on monitoring.)

 People with type 1 diabetes need to test at least before meals and at bedtime because their blood glucose level determines their dose of insulin. People who have stable type 2 diabetes may test once or twice a day.

Devout Dieting

If you are what you eat, then you have the choice of being controlled or uncontrolled depending upon what you put into your mouth. If you gain weight, you gain insulin resistance, but a small amount of weight loss can reverse the situation.

The main point you should understand about a "diabetic diet" is that it's a healthy diet for anyone, whether they have diabetes or not. You shouldn't feel like a social outcast because you're eating the right foods. You don't need special supplements; the diet is balanced and contains all the vitamins and minerals you require (although you want to be sure you're getting enough calcium).

You can follow a diabetic diet wherever you are, not just at home. Every menu has something on it that's appropriate for you.

Tenacious Testing

 The people who make smoke detectors recommend that you change the battery without fail each time you have a birthday. You should use the same simple device to remember your "complication detectors." Make sure that your doctor checks your urine for tiny amounts of protein and your feet for loss of sensation every year around the time of your birthday.

It takes five to ten years to develop complications of diabetes. When you know the problem is present, you can do a lot to slow it down or even reverse it. Never has it been truer that "an ounce of prevention is worth a pound of cure."

I make it very easy for you to get the tests you need at the time you need them. Chapter 3 gives you the current testing recommendations. Demand that you get the tests when they are due. A doctor with a busy medical practice may forget whether you have had the tests you need, but you don't have an excuse for forgetting.

Enthusiastic Exercising

When you take insulin (as opposed to pills), controlling your diabetes is a little harder because you have to coordinate your food intake and the activity of the insulin. But I have patients who've had diabetes for decades and have little trouble balancing their food and insulin. They are the enthusiastic exercisers. They use exercise to burn up glucose in place of insulin. The result is a much more narrow range of blood glucose levels than is true of the insulin takers who do not exercise. They also have more leeway in their diet because the exercise makes up for slight excesses.

I'm not talking about an hour of running each day or 50 miles on the bike. Moderate exercise like brisk walking can accomplish the same thing. The key is to exercise faithfully.

Lifelong Learning

So much is going on in the field of diabetes that I have trouble keeping up with it, and it's my specialty. How can you expect to know when doctors come up with the major advances that will cure your diabetes? The answer is lifelong learning.

After you get past the shock of the diagnosis, you're ready to learn. This book contains a lot of basic stuff that you need to know. You can even take a good course in diabetes. Then you need to keep learning. Go to meetings of the local diabetes association. Become a member of the American Diabetes Association and get its terrific magazine called *Diabetes Forecast.*

Remember that a lot of misinformation is available on the Web, so you must be careful to check out a recommendation before you start to follow it. Even information on reliable sites may not be right for your particular problem.

Above all, never stop learning! The next thing you learn may be the one that will cure you.

Meticulous Medicating

Compliance, which means treating your disease in accordance with your doctor's instructions, is a term that has special relevance for the patient with a chronic disease like diabetes who must take medications day in and day out. Sure, it's a pain (even if you could take insulin by mouth and not by injection). But the basic assumption is that you're taking your medication. Your doctor bases all his or her decisions on that assumption. Some very serious mistakes can be made if that assumption is false.

Every time a study is done on why patients' health conditions do not improve, compliance is high up on (and often leads) the list of reasons. Do you make a conscious decision to skip your pills, or do you forget?

 The best thing to do is to set up a system so that you're forced to remember. Keeping your pills in a dated container quickly shows you if you have taken them or not. You might even divide the pills by time of day.

Appropriate Attitude

Your approach to your disease can go a long way toward determining whether you will live in diabetes heaven or diabetes hell. If you have a positive attitude, treating diabetes as a challenge and an opportunity, not only is it easier for you to manage your disease, but your body actually produces chemicals that make it happen. A negative attitude, on the other hand, results in the kind of pessimism that leads to failure to diet, failure to exercise, and failure to take your medications. Plus, your body makes chemicals that are bad for you.

Diabetes is a challenge because you have to think about doing certain things that others never have to worry about. It brings out the quality of organization, which can then be transferred to other parts of your life. When you're organized, you accomplish much more in less time.

Diabetes is an opportunity because it forces you to make healthy choices for your diet as well as your exercise. You may end up a lot healthier than your neighbor without diabetes. As you make more and more healthy choices, you feel and test less and less like a person with diabetes.

Preventive Planning

Life is full of surprises. Like the sign on a display of "I Love You Only" Valentine cards: Available in Multipacks. You never know when you'll get more than you bargained for. That's why having a plan to deal with the unexpected is so important.

Say you're invited to someone's home, and they serve something that you know will raise your blood glucose significantly. What do you do? Or you go out to eat and are given a menu of incredible choices, many of which are just not for you. How do you handle that? You run into great stress at work or at home. Do you allow it to throw off your diet, your exercise, and your medication-taking?

The key to these situations is the realization that it's not possible for everything to go right all the time. In the case of the friend who cooked the wrong thing for you, eat a small portion to limit the damage. At the restaurant, you should come prepared with the food choices you know will keep you on your diet. It may be better not to look at the menu and simply discuss with your waiter what is available from your list of correct foods. And if you allow stress to throw you off, you add the problems of poor diabetic control to your other stress, making it considerably worse.

Consider doing dry runs to prepare for potentially difficult situations. For example, if you've been invited to a new restaurant, visit it in advance and simply read the menu. Carefully select the foods that will help you to stay in control. Practicing handling these situations before they arise makes it a lot easier to function when you are faced with the real thing.

Fastidious Foot Care

A recent headline read: "Hospital sued by seven foot doctors." I would certainly not like to treat any doctor with seven feet or even a doctor who is seven feet tall. Whether you have two feet or seven feet, you must take good care of them. The problem occurs when you can't feel with your feet because of neuropathy. You can easily know when this problem exists just by checking with a 10-gram filament. (Chapter 3 tells you where to get one.) If your feet cannot feel the filament, they will not feel burning hot water, a stone, a nail in your shoe, or an infected ulcer of your foot.

When you lose sensation in your feet, your eyes must replace the pain fibers that would otherwise tell you there's a problem. Carefully examine your feet every day. Your doctor should inspect your feet at every visit.

Diabetes is the primary source of foot amputations, but this drastic situation is entirely preventable if you pay attention to your feet. Test bath water by hand, shake your shoes out before you put them on, wear new shoes only a short while before checking for pressure spots, get a 10-gram filament and see whether you can feel it. The future of your feet is in your hands.

The other aspect of fastidious foot care is making sure the circulation in the blood vessels of your feet remains open. This is done by your doctor performing an ankle-brachial index. This test should be done once a year and quickly tells you and your doctor if you're experiencing a problem with your circulation.

Essential Eye Care

You're reading this book, which means you are seeing this book. So far, there are no plans to put out a Braille edition, so you had better take care of your eyes or you will miss out on the wonderful gems of information that brighten every page.

Caring for your eyes starts with a careful examination by an ophthalmologist or optometrist. You need to have an exam at least once a year. If you have controlled your diabetes meticulously, the doctor will find two normal eyes. If not, signs of diabetic eye disease may show up. At that point, you need to control your diabetes, which means controlling your blood glucose. You also want to control your blood pressure because high blood pressure contributes to worsening eye disease, as does high cholesterol.

Although the final word is not in on the effects of smoking and excessive alcohol on eye disease in diabetes, is it worth risking your sight for another puff of a cigarette? Even at this later stage, you can stop the progression of the eye disease or reverse some of the damage if you stop smoking now.

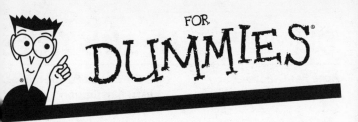

What makes **For Dummies** *Health titles so popular?*

Whenever a condition is diagnosed, people need fast, easy-to-understand answers.

Readers get the essential information on treatments, medications, and lifestyle changes. They'll also find out how to begin and maintain an exercise program and stick to healthy eating habits.

Our health titles feature:
- Expert authors with excellent credentials. In fact – many of our authors still work daily in the medical profession

- Content that can be used by both the patient and caregiver

- Local editions where applicable

- A comprehensive approach to treating or managing the condition – from medications to diet and exercise

DUMMIES ᶠᵒᴿ *Health Titles*

Acne For Dummies
978-0-471-74698-0 • 312 pp.
$16.99 US • $21.99 CAN • £11.99 UK

AD/HD For Dummies
978-0-7645-3712-7 • 356 pp.
$19.99 US • $25.99 CAN • £13.99 UK

Alzheimer's For Dummies
978-0-7645-3899-5 • 384 pp.
$21.99 US • $31.99 CAN • £14.99 UK

**Arthritis For Dummies,
2nd Edition**
978-0-7645-7074-2 • 380 pp.
$19.99 US • $25.99 CAN • £13.99 UK

**Arthritis For Dummies,
UK Edition**
978-0-470-02582-6 • 400 pp.
£14.99 UK

Asthma For Dummies
978-0-7645-4233-6 • 380 pp.
$19.99 US • $25.99 CAN • £12.99 UK

**Asthma & Allergies For
Dummies, Australian Edition**
978-1-74031-054-3 • 272 pp.
$39.95 AUS

**Back Pain Remedies For
Dummies**
978-0-7645-5132-1 • 384 pp.
$19.99 US • $25.99 CAN • £14.99 UK

Breast Cancer For Dummies
978-0-7645-2482-0 • 384 pp.
$21.99 US • $28.99 CAN • £15.50 UK

**Breast Cancer For Dummies,
Australian Edition**
978-1-74031-143-4 • 376 pp.
$39.95 AUS

**The Calorie Counter For
Dummies**
978-0-470-56834-7 • 448 pp.
$7.99 US • $9.99 CAN • £5.99 UK

**The Calorie Counter Journal
For Dummies**
978-0-470-63998-6 • 448 pp.
$12.99 US • £12.99 UK

Celiac Disease For Dummies
978-0-470-16036-7 • 384 pp.
$19.99 US • $23.99 CAN

**Chemotherapy and
Radiation For Dummies**
978-0-7645-7832-8 • 380 pp.
$21.99 US • $28.99 CAN • £13.99 UK

**Chronic Fatigue Syndrome
For Dummies**
978-0-470-11772-9 • 384 pp.
$21.99 US • $25.99 CAN • £14.99 UK

Chronic Pain For Dummies
978-0-471-75140-3 • 384 pp.
$19.99 US • $25.99 CAN • £13.99 UK

**Complementary Medicine
For Dummies, UK Edition**
978-0-470-02625-0 • 448 pp.
£15.99 UK

Conquering Childhood Obesity For Dummies
978-0-471-79146-1 • 338 pp.
$19.99 US • $25.99 CAN • £13.99 UK

Controlling Cholesterol For Dummies
978-0-7645-5440-7 • 360 pp.
$21.99 US • $28.99 CAN • £16.50 UK

COPD For Dummies
978-0-470-24757-0 • 338 pp.
$19.99 US • $21.99 CAN • £13.99 UK

Cosmetic Surgery For Dummies
978-0-7645-7835-9 • 382 pp.
$21.99 US • $30.99 CAN • £14.99 UK

Diabetes Cookbook For Dummies, 3rd Edition
978-0-470-53644-5 • 392 pp.
$19.99 US • $23.99 CAN

Diabetes Cookbook For Dummies, UK Edition
978-0-470-51219-7 • 384 pp.
£15.99 UK

Diabetes For Canadians For Dummies, 2nd Edition
978-0-470-15677-3 • 408 pp.
$29.99 CAN

Diabetes For Dummies, 3rd Edition
978-0-470-27086-8 • 408 pp.
$21.99 US

Diabetes For Dummies, 2nd Australian Edition
978-1-74031-094-9 • 544 pp.
$39.95 AUS

Diabetes For Dummies, 2nd UK Edition
978-0-470-05810-7 • 396 pp.
£15.99 UK

Eating Disorders For Dummies
978-0-470-22549-3 • 364 pp.
$19.99 US • $21.99 CAN • £13.99 UK

Endometriosis For Dummies
978-0-470-05047-7 • 362 pp.
$21.99 US • $25.99 CAN • £14.99 UK

Fertility & Infertility For Dummies, UK Edition
978-0-470-05750-6 • 384 pp.
£15.99 UK

Fibromyalgia For Dummies, 2nd Edition
978-0-470-14502-9 • 360 pp.
$21.99 US • $28.99 CAN • £16.50 UK

Food Allergies For Dummies
978-0-470-09584-3 • 384 pp.
$19.99 US • $23.99 CAN • £13.99 UK

Gluten-Free Cooking For Dummies
978-0-470-17810-2 • 342 pp.
$19.99 US • $21.99 CAN • £13.99 UK

DUMMIES *Health Titles*

The Glycemic Index Diet For Dummies
978-0-470-53870-8 • 384 pp.
$19.99 US • $23.99 CAN • £14.99 UK

Hair Loss & Replacement For Dummies
978-0-470-08787-9 • 336 pp.
$16.99 US • $18.99 CAN • £11.99 UK

Healing Foods For Dummies
978-0-7645-5198-7 • 352 pp.
$19.99 US • $27.99 CAN • £14.99 UK

Healthy Aging For Dummies
978-0-470-14975-1 • 384 pp.
$21.99 US • $25.99 CAN • £14.99 UK

The Healthy Heart Cookbook For Dummies
978-0-7645-5222-9 • 384 pp.
$19.99 US • $27.99 CAN • £14.99 UK

Heart Disease For Dummies
978-0-7645-4155-1 • 384 pp.
$19.99 US • $23.99 CAN • £12.99 UK

Heartburn & Reflux For Dummies
978-0-7645-5688-3 • 360 pp.
$19.99 US • $25.99 CAN • £13.99 UK

Herbal Remedies For Dummies
978-0-7645-5127-7 • 384 pp.
$21.99 US • $25.99 CAN • £16.50 UK

High Blood Pressure For Dummies, 2nd Edition
978-0-470-13751-2 • 360 pp.
$21.99 US • $25.99 CAN • £16.50 UK

Hypoglycemia For Dummies 2nd Edition
978-0-470-12170-2 • 288 pp.
$16.99 US • $21.99 CAN • £12.95 UK

IBS Cookbook For Dummies
978-0-470-53072-6 • 360 pp.
$21.99 US • $25.99 CAN • £15.99 UK

IBS For Dummies
978-0-7645-9814-2 • 384 pp.
$19.99 US • $23.99 CAN • £12.99 UK

IBS For Dummies, UK Edition
978-0-470-51737-6 • 402 pp.
£15.99 UK

Infertility For Dummies
978-0-470-11518-3 • 362 pp.
$21.99 US • $25.99 CAN

Living Dairy-Free For Dummies
978-0-470-63316-8 • 384 pp.
$19.99 US • $23.99 CAN • £14.99 UK

Living Gluten-Free For Dummies, 2nd Edition
978-0-470-58589-4 • 384 pp.
$19.99 US • $23.99 CAN

DUMMIES *Health Titles*

Living Gluten-free For Dummies, Australian Edition
978-0-731-40760-6 • 200 pp.
$34.95 AUS

Living Gluten Free For Dummies, UK Edition
978-0-470-31910-9 • 384 pp.
€15.99 UK

Living With Hepatitis C For Dummies
978-0-7645-7620-1 • 312 pp.
$16.99 US • $19.99 CAN • £11.99 UK

Low-Cholesterol Cookbook For Dummies
978-0-7645-7160-2 • 384 pp.
$19.99 US • $25.99 CAN

Low-Cholesterol Cookbook For Dummies, UK Edition
978-0-470-71401-0 • 384 pp.
£15.99 UK

Macrobiotics For Dummies
978-0-470-40138-5 • 384 pp.
$19.99 US •$21.99 CAN • £13.99 UK

Managing PCOS For Dummies, UK Edition
978-0-470-05794-0 • 376 pp.
£15.99 UK

Medical Ethics For Dummies
978-0-470-87856-9• 384 pp.
$24.99 US • $29.99 CAN • £17.99 UK

Medical Terminology For Dummies
978-0-470-27965-6 • 384 pp.
$21.99 US • $23.99 CAN • £14.99 UK

Medicare Prescription Drugs For Dummies
978-0-470-27676-1 • 384 pp.
$19.99 US • $21.99 CAN • £10.99 UK

Menopause For Dummies, 2nd Edition
978-0-470-05343-0 • 384 pp.
$21.99 US • $25.99 CAN

Menopause For Dummies, Australian Edition
978-1-74031-140-3 • 363 pp.
$39.95 AUS

Menopause For Dummies, UK Edition
978-0-470-06100-8 • 384 pp.
£15.99 UK

Migraines For Dummies
978-0-7645-5485-8 • 330 pp.
$19.99 US • $25.99 CAN • £14.95 UK

Multiple Sclerosis For Dummies
978-0-470-05592-2 • 362 pp.
$21.99 US • $25.99 CAN • £14.99 UK

Obsessive Compulsive Disorder For Dummies
978-0-47029331-7 • 384 pp.
$19.99 US • $21.99 CAN • £13.99 UK

DUMMIES *Health Titles*

Osteoporosis For Dummies
978-0-7645-7621-8 • 308 pp.
$16.99 US • $21.99 CAN • £11.99 UK

Parkinson's Disease For Dummies
978-0-470-07395-7 • 364 pp.
$19.99 US • $23.99 CAN • £13.99 UK

Prediabetes For Dummies
978-0-470-52301-8 • 384 pp.
$21.99 US • $25.99 CAN • £15.99 UK

Prostate Cancer For Dummies
978-0-7645-1974-1 • 384 pp.
$21.99 US • $28.99 CAN • £15.50 UK

Schizophrenia For Dummies
978-0-470-25927-6 • 384 pp.
$19.99 US • $21.99 CAN • £13.99 UK

Sleep Disorders For Dummies
978-0-7645-3901-5 • 375 pp.
$19.99 US • $25.99 CAN • £13.99 UK

Stem Cells For Dummies
978-0-470-25928-3 • 384 pp.
$21.99 US • $23.99 CAN • £14.99 UK

Stroke For Dummies
978-0-7645-7201-2 • 354 pp.
$19.99 US • $25.99 CAN • £13.99 UK

Thyroid For Dummies, 2nd Edition
978-0-471-78755-6 • 384 pp.
$19.99 US • $23.99 CAN

Thyroid For Dummies, UK Edition
978-0-470-03172-8 • 320 pp.
£15.99 UK

Treating Your Back & Neck Pain For Dummies, UK Edition
978-0-470-03599-3 • 384 pp.
£14.99 UK

Type 1 Diabetes For Dummies
978-0-470-17811-9 • 360 pp.
$21.99 US • $23.99 CAN • £14.99 UK

Understanding Autism For Dummies
978-0-7645-2547-6 • 365 pp.
$19.99 US • $23.99 CAN • £13.99 UK

Understanding Prescription Drugs For Canadians For Dummies
978-0-470-83835-8 • 384 pp.
$24.99 CAN

Vitamin D For Dummies
978-0-470-89175-9 • 288 pp.
$16.99 US • $19.99 CAN • £13.99 UK

Vitamins For Dummies
978-0-7645-5179-6 • 360 pp.
$21.99 US • $25.99 CAN • £18.99 UK

Look for these titles wherever books are sold.